Praise for *Journeying*

"This book is written in a language that I [...] language of love. This book tells the story [...] smashes the limits that the language of understanding imposes on us. In this land where this language is the native language, life and death, health and illness, hope and despair are seen in the light of the sacredness of love—the Sacred. As I read this book I felt that I was in that sacred place with them."

Wynand Johannes de Kock, Th.D.
Professor of Practical Theology,
Palmer Theological Seminary at Eastern University
Global Associate, Office of Innovation and New Ventures, Eastern University
Philadelphia, PA, and Victoria, Australia

"Dr. Robert Crick is able to reach out with courage, hope and genuine compassion to many who find themselves in the processes of grief and having a desire to overcome grief in their lives. I highly encourage and recommend every person, every couple, every pastor to own a copy of this book, which is destined to change lives of all who read it."

Bishop Krish P. Naidoo
Founder/Pastor, Destiny Prayer Chapel
Pietermaritzburg, South Africa

"Immediately, this wonderfully written book pulled me into Jeanette's story. It pricked my heart and my soul. Literally, I could not put the book down. It is powerful, inspiring, and truthful. Everyone needs to enter into this story and learn from it. Previously, I had a visceral response to the great curse called Alzheimer's. I've cried, 'God, please do not let me get that awful disease!' However, Dr. Crick has shown us how to move into it with grace and faith. The world desperately needs to know this story."

William Payne, Ph.D.
The Harlan & Wilma Hollewell Professor of Evangelism/Missions
Director of Chaplaincy Studies
Ashland Theological Seminary

"Dr. Crick and his family have given us a beautifully transparent look into their transformational journey with their beloved Jeanette into and through the world of Alzheimer's disease. This journey requires a cleansing of self-centered lifestyles and ideologies and leads to the pure revelation of the eternal relationship we have with one another and with our Abba Father. What a journey, what a struggle, what a challenge, and what a revelation."

Jeff Bower, MDiv; DVM
Owner/Veterinarian, Ark Animal Hospital
Hiram, GA

"With soul-searching honesty and courage, Bob Crick invites us to follow along as he remembers the most painful yet glorious journey of his life— the intimate sojourn with his wife Jeanette as she was forced to walk down the road of Alzheimer's disease. Bob's willingness to be led down that road has now given us an amazing map that is sure to help so many of us to find our way to the very end."

Rickie Moore, PhD
Professor of Old Testament
Lee University,
Cleveland, Tennessee

"*Journeying with Jeanette: A Love Story into the Land and Language of Alzheimer's* chronicles an exceptional love story, but it also serves as a basic introduction to the facts about Alzheimer's disease, its development, and treatment. Above all, it testifies to the amazing power of a sincere, deeply held faith in God to nurture and sustain, even in the darkest of circumstances."

Mark L. Williams, D.D.
Presiding Bishop/General Overseer
Church of God
Cleveland, Tennessee

"Dr. Robert Crick's heart has always been committed to promoting the value of others. Out of that heart comes this book that will be a treasure to all who read and especially for those journeying through their own pain. Lessons from pain have been a constant theme of his international ministry. It has never been more powerfully expressed than in the pages that follow. Be prepared to laugh, cry, reflect, and to cherish the ones you are blessed to love."

Bishop Darrell W. Waller, Ph.D.
Senior Pastor, Winchester Church of God
Winchester, VA

"Nothing I have ever read or undertaken has prepared me for the sojourn that *Journeying with Jeanette: A Love Story into the Land and Language of Alzheimer's* would take me on. Robert Crick's memoire of his beloved life-partner's final years is an extraordinary story of internal spiritual migration. This is a spiritual classic for the ages."

Dale T. Irvin, PH.D.
President and Professor of World Christianity
New York Theological Seminary
New York, NY

"This book took me with Robert Crick as he learned to listen to Jeanette's heart and her love for God as she progressed in her Alzheimer's. Dr. Crick wrote the book, but it is Jeanette's story. I am going to use the wisdom of these pages as a model for family life, especially to those in crisis, and I look forward to sharing it with others involved in pastoral care."

Bishop Calvin Eastham, MDiv
Chaplain (LTC), US Army Retired
Oklahoma City, OK

"This is an astounding narrative of a couple who suffered together through a relentless disease, Alzheimer's. Their testimony reaffirms that He is in control even in the midst of our struggles against seemingly daunting conditions in our lives and never fails to elevate His children's faith when they persist in trusting Him."

Kye Kim, M.D.
Geriatric Psychiatrist and Professor
Virginia Tech Carilion School of Medicine
Roanoke, VA

"Dr. Robert Crick weaves as one on a mission, to integrate head, heart, and hands in a volume dedicated not only to Alzheimer's Dementia as an illness with clinical and pastoral needs, but one with a personal face and personal story. I am moved as a person by the narrative pathos of this work, provoked as a clinician by the psycho-social-emotional dialogue of *Journeying with Jeanette*, and inspired as a pastor to offer comprehensive care to move from 'freedom from' to 'freedom to' a Holy God in the context of human frailty."

Patrick Jenson, MD
Psychiatry and Senior Pastor
Cary, NC

"As the father of a child with autism, I read Dr. Crick's book nodding, wiping away tears, and finally, absorbing its timely message about human dignity and the value of people with special needs. With his beautiful love story that is so much more, Dr. Crick teaches us not to feel sorry for such people or to try to 'fix' them, but to learn from them and to understand their indispensable role in God's plan for the world and for each of us."

Joseph E. Viviano, J.S.D.
Viviano Law
Vivano, Pagano & Howlett, PLLC
Mt. Clemens, Michigan

"As an activities professional who has worked for over twenty years with the Alzheimer's population, I highly recommend Dr. Crick's new book, *Journeying with Jeanette*. It is this personal story that enabled her medical team to acknowledge her as a person rather than just someone to be taken care of. It is a must read for anyone who desires to work with the Alzheimer's population."

Margie Henry, Activity Consultant Certified
Heritage of Sandy Plains
Marietta, GA

"I highly recommend this book to those people who are dealing with Alzheimer's and the many other types of loss. Dr. Robert Crick's openness regarding his pain and his struggle to deal with Jeanette's sickness and death provides valuable insights for students, patients, and family members. I also recommend it to those who want to learn not only about Alzheimer's, but about being human, facing loss, and the struggle to trust one's God on such a path."

Keith Munford, D.Min.
ACPE Supervisor, Adjunct Professor and Hospice Chaplain
Chattanooga, TN

"For pastors and families who have loved ones afflicted with this incurable disease, this book is a goldmine of insight, passion and Christian ministry. With Alzheimer's disease being the third leading cause of death among our senior citizens, spiritual caregivers must educate themselves about the needs of this growing population within our congregations and neighborhoods."

Charles Howell, M. Div.
MOAA Chaplain
Chaplain (Colonel), US Army (Ret.)
Augusta, GA

"*Journeying with Jeanette* is the story of how the Crick family faced and overcame the horrible vicissitudes of dealing with diagnosis and progression of Alzheimer's disease in their beloved wife and mother by developing a person-oriented model of care that provided support and comfort for Jeanette and her family. It emphasizes the role of family, a personalized model of care, and for the Cricks, the role of their deeply held faith."

Mark Frankel, MD
Psychiatry
Cleveland, OH

"*Journeying with Jeanette* is more than a novel, a family experience, or another book. Dr. Crick offers the paradigm for overcoming life struggles, suffering, sufficiency, and sorrows. The powerful message that comes across the book is that human suffering and death cannot destroy the faith, the hope, and the divine potential of a life well lived."

Radu Tirle, D. Min.
Former Romanian Congressional Senator and Regional President
Professor, Pentecostal Theological Institute
Bucharest, Romania

JOURNEYING
with Jeanette

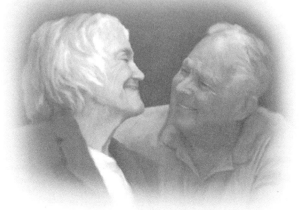

JOURNEYING
with Jeanette

A Love Story into the Land and Language of
ALZHEIMER'S

ROBERT CRICK

with Brandelan Miller

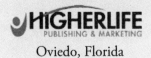

Oviedo, Florida

Journeying with Jeanette: A Love Story into the Land and Language of Alzheimer's

by Robert Crick, DMin, Supervisor, ACPE

Published by

HigherLife Publishing & Marketing, Inc.

PO Box 623307

Oviedo, Florida 32762

www.ahigherlife.com

Paperback ISBN: 978-1-939183-97-2

ebook ISBN: 978-1-939183-98-9

Cover Design: Bill Johnson

First Edition

16 17 18 19 20 21 — 9 8 7 6 5 4 3 2 1

Printed in the United States of America

"The King will reply, 'Truly I tell you, whatever you did for one of the least of these brothers and sisters of mine, you did for me.'"

—Matthew 25: 40 (NIV)

Table of Contents

Foreword

by Brandelan Miller

This book is the second project I have had the pleasure and honor to work on with Dr. Robert Crick. Without a doubt, this project was the most personal. My initial interest was our shared desire to give families with special or medical needs a platform within the church they need and deserve. (I believe this book will, at least, start that conversation going forward.) What I didn't expect was the profound impact this book would have on my immediate life. While Alzheimer's is the central topic lifted up, we can all relate to loss, fear of loss, major life transitions, identity crises, and the need to make all of life, God, and faith fit into our "control box." To be honest, I was terribly afraid to assist in the development of this book. It is far outside my normal writing assignments. But God has a way of preparing us—even putting us in places which make the emotions of the text come alive in our own lives, albeit in unique and trying ways.

I could not have known, from the first month we started this project to its end, that my life would be thrown into a major transition. With that transition came loss, fear, issues of identity, and the need for something familiar to anchor my disoriented and embattled heart. Assisting the Cricks in the writing of their story opened a door for me to actively process those feelings and perceptions.

1

Often, Dr. Crick would call weeping after I submitted my work on a chapter. He would state that he couldn't understand how I knew what they experienced, how they felt. Our vision was short in those early months. How could I possibly know what it is like to sacrifice your heart and life for the one you love due to Alzheimer's Disease? How could I know the identity crisis that takes place in the midst of those transitions or the pain of losing someone in a most horrifying way? The reality is we all do. We all know these experiences—maybe not in the specifics, but certainly in the generic. And so, when Dr. Crick experienced losing Jeanette, I knew the powerful and paralyzing life moments of losing a person to a disease that was so unkind. In 2006, my younger cousin, who had been struggling with severe depression and drug abuse, took his life in my basement on New Year's morning as I was getting ready for church. Every moment was a lifetime; no moment was real; everything was outside of me. While I had the privilege of writing about Dr. Crick's immediate moments (to include the funeral), much of what I wrote was my own experience superimposed on his. Yet, as he later explained, so true to his own.

I fully understood what it meant to give up a life you loved and exchange it for something costly and taxing so that the person you love most in this world would find their greatest known purpose. Jeanette found that purpose as Alzheimer's liberated her heart to meet Jesus like a little child—welcomed and free; and my husband in making the difficult decision to be liberated from the corporate world for the sacrificial and fearful work of full-time ministry in a place many hours from the people we know and love. Like Dr.

Crick—through different pathways—I know what it is like to have to rethink my role, give up old identities and purposes for a role that seems remedial, minimal, insignificant...only to discover a new a profound understanding of God and self.

Many times I thought we would never finish this book. Life kept getting in the way. Dr. Crick would say to me, "Sunny, let me know if it is too much for you. I know your life is chaotic right now. I care too much about you to let you be overwhelmed by the task of writing this book."

Was it overwhelming? Yes, at times. But, it was also my lifeline. As is often the case in life, his story was my story. His testimony then became my saving grace as I was forced to answer the question over and over, "Where is God in our stories?" The constant and repeated answer that anchored me then and continues to anchor me today, that was echoed on every page of this book, is that God is in every detail of our stories. He is not hidden from us, if we choose to see Him there. Is He always the delivering God? I WISH, but no. Rather, He is always, without fail, a covenanting God who is with us, for us, and always toward us. This book didn't change me; instead it gifted me with the arduous task of persevering—at times with great resistance—in faith, in hope, and in love as I confronted my own suffering, daily. In so doing, it became my entry way into Dr. Crick's story. I suppose, without knowing it, the Lord was allowing me the privilege of an incarnate ministry. That is, by entering in to my own pain, I could fully engage his and vice versa. For this was certainly a mutual experience of grace, healing, and hope...as I believe it will be for anyone who enters the story with us.

Acknowledgments

Of course, those closest to Jeanette and me, who gave us the most support in our long, painful, tedious, yet victorious journey into the land and language of Alzheimer's, were our kids and grandkids: including our oldest son, David, his wife, Robyn, their three kids, Samantha, Mackenzie, and Dylan; our daughter, Jonne; and, our son, Dale, his wife, Carmen, and their children, Rachel and Jonah. As you will discover in this book, all of my kids and their families were active participants in every phase of Jeanette's journey with Alzheimer's, from the earliest symptoms until that time we joined together around the bedside to say goodbye to a wonderful wife, mother, and "Oma."

Special thanks go, as well, to our extended families on both Jeanette's side (Lees) as well as mine (Cricks). Geri, Jeanette's younger sister, represented the best of Jeanette's extended family's love and care. Jeanette expected this close relationship, and it was apparent right up to her death. Then, on my side, the "Crick clan," I want to express my special thanks for the love and prayers given daily by my many nieces and nephews. My niece, Mary Massey, a.k.a. "my Blossom," who was more like my younger sister, represented the best of this other large family connection. Since I was the "last" of the original group of 16 brothers and sisters, my loss of

5

Jeanette reminded me that the patriarchs of the Crick heritage were passing off the scene and that more than ever they must draw closer together, loving and caring, as if there may be no tomorrow.

This book, as well as my earlier one, *Outside the Gates: Theology, History and Practice of Chaplaincy Ministries*, was co-researched and written with my ministry colleague, Brandelan Miller. My special thanks go to her for not just her unique academic and ministry skills, but the passions of her call to make sure that those with these special needs are genuinely valued as "persons, not clients," and are given a prominent place at the tables of our local church ministry endeavors.

It is impossible for me to list all those who stood by Jeanette and me as we journeyed together toward the land of Alzheimer's. Having been together for 66 years in life and in ministry, obviously we accumulated hundreds of friends and colleagues around the world. Both the individuals and groups mentioned poured their best loving care into us, which gave us the strength to not only sustain Alzheimer's but to learn some of God's most precious lessons as a result of it.

Besides our immediate family, it was our "chaplaincy family" who stood the closest by us in our battles and victories in dealing with Alzheimer's. Chaplains, by their very nature, go where the pain is the greatest. They were with us in joy and tears, letters, telephone calls, emails addressed to "My Spiritual Mom," and especially toward the end, sharing my family's grief with intense love and support. I would love to mention all of them by name, and yet, we are talking about hundreds: chaplains representing ministry in the military, prisons, hospitals, industries, college/university campuses, and more than a thousand volunteer chaplains trained through our Commission representing many countries. This special chaplaincy love and care relationship with this unique group of caregivers goes back for Jeanette and me more than 50 years. Naturally, a book of this nature should be dedicated to those who spend their lives in crises situations, what we call "ministry beyond the gates," not because they got stuck there, but because love and care at these intense levels are part of their DNA.

Then, there are all those other special relationships, other associations of a "special order:" our Seminary colleagues and students, led by President Lamar Vest, pastors, CPE fellow supervisors, and, what proved to be so needed, my counseling clients. My appreciation also goes to the River of Life Church of God, Cumming, GA, whose pastoral staff and members provided for Jeanette and me a genuine safe haven as we faced the most critical issues of life.

We could not have made this Alzheimer's journey together without the many outstanding professional, medical, and various care agencies and personnel. My deepest gratitude go especially to the medical staffs of Emory University Hospital's Wesley Woods Clinic, whose initial evaluations taught us to take charge of our medical and care needs, and not to depend upon someone else's prescribed "one fits all" model. With that freedom, we discovered Dr. Scott Cooper, a local neurologist, about halfway through our Alzheimer's journey. His practical, down-to-earth approach as "more coach than player" enabled us to design a family program that moved Jeanette from being just another "client" toward that of a "person." Our other back-up, home care was primarily with our local Comfort Keeper agency, who supplied us with many home caregivers for nearly three years—all good, but three who were especially "just right" for the two of us. Brittany Sizemore and Kasea Zeamer, were probably the youngest of our many caregivers. They saw and treated Jeanette as if she was their mom or grandmother. Jeanette adored them. And then, Jasman Dennis, who expressed love, passion and care as if it was her Christian call and ministry. Thank God for the many caregivers, making minimum salaries, but giving maximum heart and soul care.

Finally, I must lift up those who were not only friends, but my spiritual dialogue partners, reflecting with me at a deep personal level throughout this long Alzheimer's journey and the writing of this book. First, let me highlight those directly connected to the sponsor of this book, The Outside the Gates Foundation. Paul and Rhonda Stockard, our chaplaincy trainers for Africa, were always there when our pain was the most intense. Dr. Jimmy Dupree, an Outside the Gates founding board member, whose mother struggled and died with Alzheimer's, gave good, level-headed insight into the daily twist and turns of caring for Jeanette. Elaine Offutt, another board member, and her late husband, Tom, helped develop and finance Outside the Gates Ministries right up to the printing of this new book. Her own long battles with various illnesses and surgeries never hindered her daily prayers for me and Jeanette— prayers so needed and so timely.

Of course, there are so many others. Dr. Steven Land, former President of our Seminary, now professor in the area of Pentecostal Theology, was never out of touch with our pain, especially our need to look deeply into the Scriptures in regards to what this battle, with its many losses and victories, was doing to our souls. Dr. Rickie Moore, equally, was there with me as the Alzheimer's journey took me and my family deeper into its dark waters. His daughter, Hannah, in her long journey with a crippling disease, and yet with a driving passion for a full, productive life and ministry, became the means by which we could minister and theologically reflect as "wounded healers."

Those mentioned represent hundreds who travelled with us through sickness, family development, occupational successes and struggles, and in the development of this book. In preparing for our journey into the land and language of Alzheimer's, naturally, we sought out prayer and care partners…and these mentioned are but a few, representing what the Bible calls in Hebrews 12: 1-2 (NIV) "The Great Cloud of Witnesses":

"Therefore, since we are surrounded by such a great cloud of witnesses, let us throw off everything that hinders and the sin that so easily entangles, and let us run with perseverance the race marked out for us. Let us fix our eyes on Jesus, the author and perfecter of our faith, who for the joy set before him endured the cross, scorning its shame, and sat down at the right hand of the throne of God."

Introduction

The Public & Private Face of Alzheimer's Disease: Katherine Jeanette Crick

"The King will reply, 'Truly I tell you,
whatever you did for one of the least of these
brothers and sisters of mine, you did for me.'"
—Matthew 25: 40 (NIV)

In January of 2011, Katherine Jeanette Crick, my wife and life partner, was diagnosed with Alzheimer's disease. Although she was already experiencing many of the symptoms caused by the disease, we were not yet prepared to receive a diagnosis of Alzheimer's. In hind sight, there were signs everywhere. She had changed, too. We were just too busy to see what was so visible, so obvious. That didn't last long, though. Life after her diagnosis brought more changes. These changes were so great and so quick that, at times, my family and I could hardly keep up. Maybe because we had become residents of our lives rather than journeymen— nomads—being led through this great journey called life. We soon realized *residency* would not fit with the life of Alzheimer's patients.

These patients, Jeanette included, have been called to a journey—a journey that would lead them into unexpected and foreign places. Once we understood this we were able to stop struggling to keep her where we needed her and were able to release her to guide us to the places God needed all of us to go. Our journey required a great commitment on our part to faithfully care for her no matter what that might look like. Over time it became a commitment to travel closely with her as she led us toward her purposed destination, *the land and language of Alzheimer's disease*. Of course, the greater story isn't in her destination but the transformational journey the Lord would lead us on to get there. That is where her unique face, her distinct story, emerges from the indistinct masses imprisoned by the public face of Alzheimer's disease.

The Public Face of Alzheimer's Disease

The public face of Alzheimer's disease is that part experienced through medical and other professional care agencies. It speaks to the disease alone: the various expressions of the disease through its many phases and symptoms shared by the 5.3 million persons who are currently diagnosed.[1] Our initial loss of Jeanette to that larger, global picture is what caused me to fight for her more private story. In the massive industry of the medical profession, faces are often (unintentionally) exchanged for patient numbers and manageable symptoms. I wanted her to be seen and valued, but they couldn't see

---

1 Alzheimer's Association, "2015 Alzheimer's Disease Facts and Figures," Alzheimer's & Dementia 2015, accessed December 2015, www.alz.org/facts/.

her through the mass of faces before them. She already lost so much. I wasn't going to allow her to lose herself to the "machine" of medicine. While our experience with the medical profession was troubling, the problem wasn't the public face. The public face had a necessary role. As our lives took a major detour into the many unknowns of the disease, it helped to navigate us through the complex and overwhelming world of Alzheimer's. It cautioned us to what was ahead and provided insight for present and past occurrences. Without it we would not have been able to create an effective care strategy or establish values that would be non-negotiable in more difficult times. Even things that could be predicted were overwhelming to consider, particularly for Jeanette. What we could predict were a series of phases[2] (early, middle and late) which the mind, and then body, would undergo as the disease progressed, physically attacking brain cells. Initially, this attack occurred in very minor ways: losing car keys, forgetting a face, etc. However, as the disease advanced, these minor issues became major. Eventually the nerve cells in the cerebral hemispheres of the brain (the place of logic and intellect) die. Thus, Jeanette not only forgot her life, but how to function within it. Her brain forgot how to work—how to direct her body. Soon afterwards, she succumbed

> *She already lost so much. I wasn't going to allow her to lose herself to the "machine" of medicine.*

---

2 Some physicians and researchers break the phases into more specified phases, however, it seems the most agreed upon model is the three phase model identified here.

to death due to the damage. This damage was not just to the brain, but to all other vital organs dependent on normal brain functions.

The good news is, with millions being diagnosed each year, our nation and nations around the world are finally waking up to the catastrophic possibilities of Alzheimer's disease, not just on those diagnosed but on their families and their finances. The task of caring for Jeanette was daunting. If not for the grace of God leading and directing us personally and financially, we could not have done so. Both the time invested in her daily care and the cost to carry it out would have ended our efforts. Some researchers suggest that families and other unpaid caregivers (friends, church volunteers, etc.) provide an estimate of more than 1,100 hours of unpaid care per worker every year (approximately 22 hours per week).[3] This is in addition to their normal work schedules, care of their families, and other responsibilities of life. My children's efforts in assisting me truly allowed for Jeanette to live out her days at home. But I know this act of service came with such a heavy burden to bear. When this kind of extensive care becomes too much, families look outside the home—as did my family—for additional resources. However, the cost to keep one at home, with around the clock care, comes to an

---

3 Alzheimer's Association, "2015 Alzheimer's Disease Facts and Figures," Alzheimer's & Dementia 2015, accessed December 2015, www.alz.org/facts/.

average of $360 per day. That translates into $10,800 per month or $131,400 per year.[4]

While these facts are necessary to consider, especially as you prepare to embark on this journey with your loved one, they are not the most important detail to take with you on your journey. The most important fact is this: our entire Christian faith is built on the premise that when we make our way to an altar and give our lives to Christ, from that moment forward we are in a process that will be orchestrated by our heavenly Father if we so allow it. That journey (regardless of the circumstances—Alzheimer's, cancer, or just the normal business of life) can be the most transformational experience of our lives. This is true not because of who we are, but whose we are. This, among so many other reasons, is why this is not just another "public face" event but something so special that it lines up with those mystical events in Scripture that are listed as transformative. This transformation not only occurs in spite of the disease. It happens because God, as the author and finisher of our stories, allows for the disease (this and others) to form and inform our lives in meaningful ways. This was the case with my precious Jeanette. Her story didn't end with the diagnosis; it's not even two separate testaments, Pre- and Post-Alzheimer's. Rather, her journey continues to be written even as her life chapters are being retold,

---

4 Some researchers believe the cost to the taxpayers and to the caregivers over the next few years will eventually reach hundreds of billions annually. Alzheimer's Association, "2015 Alzheimer's Disease Facts and Figures," Alzheimer's & Dementia 2015, accessed December 2015, www.alz.org/facts/.

evaluated, integrated into our own stories, and ultimately, transforming willing participants.

When an event of this magnitude happens, it absolutely makes a difference under whose orders you are traveling and whether those orders are about life, death, or the "beyond." So when the Lord directs you to get your affairs in order, this doesn't just mean the practical business of life, although that is important. He means come to the table; listen for His guidance, ready yourself for the journey, but pack light!

The Private Face of Alzheimer's Disease

The private face of Alzheimer's disease looks beyond the stats and patient numbers to see clearly the individual lives and stories which house the illness, in particular, Jeanette's story and my story. Jeanette, to me, was never just a client or victim of Alzheimer's. She was a person who in spite of the disease had a history and personal story which connected her to a community of friends and family members. In other words, the private, personal face of Alzheimer's must never be lost to its detached, public face. This distinction is imperative. Because the medical field is so terribly overloaded with clientele, particularly the elderly population, people are quickly losing their individual personhood to mere numbers. Even those doctors that really have a heart for their patients simply have limited time to "see" them, acknowledge their unique history and experience with the disease, and then respond compassionately. Subsequently, the "machine" takes over driving patients, like cattle, through the process without regard for their humanity. I learned this first-hand through Jeanette's experience and decided I would not let the machine be more prominent than the person, Katherine Jeanette Crick. Like every individual with this disease, Jeanette's history was so unique that it could not and will not ever be duplicated. So I fought to maintain those identifiers of her unique personhood. I even wrote a biographical summary of her life to distribute to her physicians. Most were simply not interested in her life; others apologetically disclosed they had no time to be interested. The very nature of the machine only allowed them to be interested in the numbered days they could effectively manage until her death. Maybe my resistance to their indifference is what has inspired me to write her story. I just believe her story is too beautiful, too unique, and too important, to not be seen and valued, too. I loved all of her story, and I loved all of her. My Jeanette was like no other.

Her uniqueness is why this seventeen-year-old boy immediately fell in love with her. I loved the way she tried to blend in, but always stood out. I loved her smile, her way of telling a story, her shape and physique. I loved her integrity, her love of the Word of God, her love for her kids, her faithfulness in every task, and her unfounded, extravagant love for me. I was drawn to *her*, the person, not just another woman in a sea of women. I wasn't going to lose her *person* to the vast sea of patient identification numbers. There was more to her story than the shared symptoms and phases of Alzheimer's. Her story was one of a kind. This is why I have to believe that—because she is a child of God, redeemed by His precious blood and given hope through His resurrection and ascension—her story matters.

They all matter to God (Ps. 139:13-16 and Mt. 6:25-34), and they must matter to us (Jn. 13:34-35, 1 Jn. 3:18, and Mk 12:31). It is our privilege and duty to preserve that "one of a kind" story found in the life of each of our loved ones. I assure you, their story matters. Hence, this book is my resistance to the *machine*. It is the story of how we refused to exchange the private face of Katherine Jeanette Crick for the public face of patient no. 3402718. How? It is very simple. We decided from the beginning that our family would journey close enough with her so as not to lose her face in the crowd.

The private face is too personal and individual to lose sight of. It speaks to one's personhood which *cannot be erased* by the devastating effects of the disease. Though many professionals might disagree, I can speak to this glorious truth. Even when Jeanette didn't know exactly who she was (a child, a mother, a visitor) or the kind of person she had chosen to be, her Christ-like character and deep love for God and people was never destroyed by the devastation of Alzheimer's disease. This single fact made our journey with her possible. As we chose to remain close, though costly to us personally, the Lord unveiled wondrous truths about His enduring, covenantal love and ours. To say this journey changed our lives is a great understatement and misunderstanding of the journey. For this journey always ends in death for those committed to it, by choice or by diagnosis. Initially it cost me my life—a life I loved and cherished, a life that made sense and satisfied. Yet in its finality, the journey gave me new life—a life abundant and full of His glory. A life with renewed purpose and vision. A life transformed by the deep, merciful and compassionate love of God that teaches us to literally be all things to all the "people" that made up Jeanette's life in the end. That transformation is what is lost when the private face is exchanged for the public face of Alzheimer's disease. Thankfully the Spirit knew better than we did. Early in the process he allowed us to discern the difference between these two faces so that we might fight hard to preserve—even elevate—that most essential, private face of Jeanette's journey through the land and language of Alzheimer's disease.

The success of our "fight" rests on one very important initial decision: the decision to travel with her *covenantally* rather than *contractually*. We decided right from the beginning that the Lord was leading us through this journey. If we were to get from it what He intended for us, we had to negotiate our journey in terms of a Godly Covenant, not a contract. The Lord would require nothing less of us than this. This is how He commits to travel with us. Am I suggesting we were without a choice? No. We had a choice. We could have let Jeanette be the only one radically changed by her journey, or we could join her on the journey and be changed by it, too. We chose the latter believing this was a covenant orchestrated by the Lord for all of *us*. Therefore, we too must be transformed.

Covenanting with her was necessary, but it didn't take away the struggle. I had to struggle with those voices inside of me that spoke with such finality. And I must confess that initially I gave too much credence to that voice of pragmatism as a professional counselor and her protective husband. *How are you going to care for her around the clock at home with all those other obligations?* (Which, I admit looked so important.) Or, *Oh, I know what this is about; I taught courses on Alzheimer's. I am ahead of the pack, so we can slide through this process without any real change or learning process.* Additionally, my favorite: *this is a disease to overcome, not a journey intended to reveal who we really are and to be transformed by the intersecting of self-knowledge and the deepened knowledge of who He really is.* Then there was the Lord's voice beckoning me to make a choice: "Whose voice will you listen to?" And, "Could this voice which declared, 'Jeanette has Alzheimer's,' be the voice of the Lord?"

Don't get me wrong. I did not settle this issue immediately. My immediate comfort or appeasement came from hearing this news as the "voice of the medical world," which at that moment explained the disease in a language I thought I had already mastered. It became my security and the manager of my dissonance. I would remind myself over and over that I was equipped and trained clinically in how to respond appropriately. Yet my refrain proved powerless over my reality. Something was missing; it just didn't feel right. Then it came. That optimal moment of revelation. My epiphany. The unmistakable truth of my reality, God's reality. Appearing first as sundry thoughts, I listened as disconnected pieces—puzzle-like pieces not yet assembled—emerged in my spirit. Thoughts like: *No, you don't know what Jeanette's journey is about. You only know of its public face; you have not yet known its private face.* Or, *For once in your life, erase from you heart those presuppositions, and let Me (the Lord) take you back to school again.* Finally, *Whose voice has the power to not only give you strength to endure this journey with Jeanette, but will cleanse you and transform you in the process?* As the pieces began to take shape in my heart, I knew that this was not just about her, it was about us. I knew beyond any doubt where this disease came from and for whom it was intended: it was *our journey*, meant for both of us, our family, and all those who will eventually read this account and choose to be changed by it.

Thus the message of Jeanette's journey isn't just for our family and friends. It is a message that extends to the local church. Jeanette's journey connected us with the global reality of the millions who are facing or who will face that pronouncement: "Your loved one has Alzheimer's." They are moms and dads, 40-year-olds and seniors, common citizens and celebrities, as well as believers and non-believers. This non-discriminant group includes President Ronald Reagan, renowned women's basketball coach Pat Summit, and acclaimed singer Glen Campbell. Like Jeanette, these and millions of others had an amazing testimony of their lives, occupations, accomplishments, family and other unique attributes that deem them as more than just a *client* or *victim*. Undoubtedly, the fierce reality of this disease is the rapid rate by which it is growing. Some studies predict that while presently more than five million people in the US have been diagnosed with Alzheimer's disease, by 2050 that number could reach 13.8 million, excluding those under the age of sixty-five.[5] What does that look like up close? Someone is developing this disease approximately every sixty-seven seconds.

While the rest of the nation is waking up to this fact, our churches are still stuck in their perfected slumber. As the body of Christ, we

---

5 "2015 Alzheimer's Disease Facts and Figures," Alzheimer's Association, January 1, 2016, www.alz.org/facts/#prevalence.

must be willing to wake up and engage the lives of those touched by this and other disabling diseases (physical, mental, intellectual, and chemical) which remove and isolate whole portions of our congregations *from* the body. The entry place is awareness. The Christian community must become better informed and better equipped to offer the ministry of Christ (Matthew 25: 40-46) to these individuals and families who often experience a great disconnect during the years they care for their families. This disease is devastating to persons and families. We must create a space in our mission to not forget, to not look away, and to not deny their existence in order to maintain our stained-glass faith. In other words, we must make it our mission to look upon the pain, sit with the anguished and awkward, become active learners, and most importantly be willing to partake in whatever journey they (or God) take us on in the process.

Chapter 1

The Awakening

I thought I was prepared, but soon found out I was not. Not even close. How could anyone be ready for *that* moment? That moment my beloved Jeanette, wife of 64 years, was diagnosed with Alzheimer's disease. It was an awakening, maybe momentarily a shattering. The moments leading up to her diagnosis seemed to be endless and overwhelming while we waited. You see, in the waiting room we are confronted with all our most despairing questions, depth (or lack) of faith, deepest fears, darkest regrets, and desperate pleas for deliverance. These will either be our giants to slay or wine presses that we hide within. I was still deciding. My mind was fixed on the probability of her illness and to what extent she—we—were already immersed in this new reality. Phrases like "initial phase," "middle phase," and "final phase" took captive my thoughts as we checked into the Alzheimer's clinic, especially that final phase.

"Final phase." Having a background in clinical chaplaincy and counseling, I knew very well what *that phase* entailed. This frightening reality normally does not come in one nicely wrapped package; it grabs your attention and sinks in layer by layer. I had suspicions for a number of years before Jeanette was formally diagnosed with the disease that, indeed, she was a "victim." Hmm. The fact that I used the label "victim" in those early days exposes how narrow my understanding was concerning the long, painful, and complex journey we were about to take. Nevertheless, in spite of our suspicions, we simply did not act on them.

Sitting there in the waiting room, I reflected on the irony of the moment. You would think that I should have been well prepared for this awakening. But, the reality is that I didn't even know I needed to be awakened. I had taught courses for many years that included an understanding of the inner workings of the disease. I relayed to ministers and counselors practical, theological models meant to offer support to families and those afflicted with Alzheimer's. I had had clients over the years who came to me for clinical support as they struggled to provide care for their loved ones who had Alzheimer's. I even had a student whose grandmother was dying from Alzheimer's disease ask, "Does God ever heal someone with this or other diseases like it?" My response was the typical, academically detached response. That non-answer, answer: "Why not?" Followed with, "The bigger question is, how are *you* going to deal with Alzheimer's and other issues of this nature in your work as a counselor or minister?"

Maybe it was those detached, clinical facts which made this moment so surreal, so other-worldly yet inevitable before me. I was already in transition, yet I had not paid attention to the obvious clues. Clues that I, as a seminary professor, who was knowledgeable in this area and understood how Alzheimer's disease worked in the gradual elimination of nerve cells within the cerebral hemispheres of the brain, should have better detected. I just wasn't ready *to be prepared for* (let alone *live in*) that jarring moment when life as we had lived it began to make a radical change.

I have since realized, like so many who teach or work in this field, I had only a working knowledge of this disease, especially the personal and corporate ways this disease affects the individuals and those who care for them. I had no idea how this disease changes the entire landscape of a family's life. I didn't really understand that almost all of life's so called "normal patterns" take on different characters and characteristics. I had never considered that this disease would force caregivers to change and be transformed radically, lest they find themselves in isolation, fear, and aloneness. I didn't know it yet, but I would come to realize very quickly the necessity of making a choice to either be changed by these truths with her or leave her to navigate them alone while I provided a detached and emotionally safe, almost sacrificial service. In other words, "I will maintain my life as it is without sharing the experience of a substantive change."

In that waiting room, the awakening room, I determined the latter would never be an option for us. First, Jeanette and I had travelled many years together. In so doing, we discovered that our faith required a shared plan for both joy and pain. So from my perspective, I had no choice but to conclude this was not just her crisis, but our joint crisis. Second, my own nature of wanting to apprehend the reason for this disease, both clinically and spiritually, made me from the beginning a shared partner. I already felt as if the Lord was taking us toward something beautiful. Something radical. A concept He would later parse out and more deeply define in my heart as a "sacrament of cleansing." And so, in the waiting room— the awakening room—I discerned in my spirit that I could not let this be her journey, alone. It was ours. It had always been ours... .

> *I discerned in my spirit that I could not let this be her journey, alone. It was ours. It had always been ours.*

My mind was working overtime in search for some logical answer to the pounding issues in my head. I guess I was looking for something—a metaphor, name, phrase or other sign—to give shape to these rambling thoughts. My mind drifted back to my many years as a military chaplain,[6] particularly our many moves from one assignment to the next.

Suddenly, it hit me—a better understanding of her ordeal and what was to follow as she would proceed into her new assignment with the Lord. Lauren Kessler calls it the *Land of Alzheimer's*.[7] I experienced it larger than that. For us, it was the

---

6 During the Korean Conflict, I served for 4 years as an enlisted airman (1952 – 1956) with duty in Germany. Upon graduation from Vanderbilt Divinity School in 1961, I was commissioned as an Army Chaplain, serving 1961 – 1978. My assignments were with several Airborne units, to include the 82 Airborne Division, 8th Infantry Division in Germany, 101 Airborne Division, 173rd Airborne Brigade in Vietnam, and the Airborne School, Fort Benning, GA. I had several other military and clinical assignments at various bases in the US. I was an Airborne Master Jumper and was awarded the Bronze Star for Valor, the Legion of Merit Award, and numerous other awards and commendations.

7 Lauren Kessler, Finding Life in the Land of Alzheimer's: One Daughter's Hopeful Story (New York: Penguin Group, 2007).

land *and language* of Alzheimer's. Not only was her experience otherworldly, but that land had a language of its own that only the inhabitants truly knew. This would be her new assignment. In my spirit, I felt the Lord give new insight into our assignment. In military language, assignments were either TDY (Temporary Duty)[8] or PCS (Permanent Change of Station). The Lord prepared my heart; this would not be a TDY. TDYs were short assignments often in a combat zone. When the crisis was over, the TDY ended and the military personnel returned home. The Lord was showing me this new assignment would be a Permanent Change of Station. This would not be a combat zone to be conquered after a brief period of time. She was not returning from that land; she was journeying toward it. At that moment, suddenly the pain and grief became more than I could bear. My daughter asked what was wrong with me. I didn't answer. I was not ready to share with her this new insight. As the day wore on, it sank in deeper and deeper that she had already begun her journey into the *land and language of Alzheimer's.* PCS, not TDY.

Then and there I knew what my deepest fears were. I knew that if we were going to make the most out of our last spiritual orders given to us by the Lord Almighty, I had to find a way to be deeply involved with *her journey,* as it would be the last journey we would take together. I knew that I could not go where the Lord was sending her, but with the work of the Holy Spirit and my willingness to change, I could at least share significantly in all the confusion, loss of memories, the breakdown of her vital organs, and the

---

8 The acronym TDY literally stands for "Temporary Duty Yonder."

pain that would come toward the end. And, just maybe, with the Lord's help, I could learn enough about the land and the language of Alzheimer's to occasionally join her part of the way into this new journey. I knew it was not the Lord's will that we PCS together, but I prayed at that moment for the wisdom, strength, grace, and guidance of the Holy Spirit to be not just an observer but a participant in what would ultimately be a complete change of everything we had labeled as "normal." It may seem strange to some, but the mere acceptance of that reality—PCS, not TDY—gave me a sense of relief.

Sitting there, waiting for the series of Alzheimer's tests to begin, I occasionally reached over to give Jeanette a hug and my daughter, Jonne, a forced smile. My head was full of information on the subject, but my heart ached for an answer as to "Why me?" and more importantly, "Why Jeanette?" I was experiencing at that moment what I so often described to students as *anticipatory grief*. Anticipatory grief anticipates "bad news," while not yet knowing how bad the news is. During that time between "what is and what may be," my mind took me quickly back to events of our long history together that suddenly seemed more sacred than life itself. In doing so, I found my greatest strength in remembering how our lives became so intertwined. It was as if in this shaken emotional state, wondering what the final verdict would be, I needed to anchor myself in the memories of our earliest relationship. My mind took me back to the moment I fell in love with her when I was only seventeen. From the moment I laid eyes on her, I was hooked. For me, it was more than love at first sight. As long as I could remember,

I dreamed for someone to belong exclusively to me. Growing up poor in a family of 16 kids during the Great Depression, it seemed that every waking hour was taken up with daydreams of finding that beautiful someone I found in Jeanette. I knew our relationship and partnership in life was all ordered and orchestrated by God. But she was more than that; she was *my* special gift from the Lord.

Caught up in those blessed memories, I couldn't help but revisit the days leading up to our wedding day, August 6, 1948. After a very short romance (five weeks to be exact), we were married by a justice of the peace with our taxi driver as the primary witness. I was only 17; she was 20. I had convinced her that if she did not marry me, I would leave and take a job in California. Of course, I was deeply in love with her, so I would have done anything to get her to marry me—even lie about my age. She finally consented, so we slipped away without our parents knowing what we were doing. After the ceremony, Jeanette called her older sister to pass the word on to her parents. When we returned from our honeymoon, our parents were furious with us for doing such a foolish thing. I have never before or since experienced the tongue lashing I got from Jeanette's dad. After he finished, he simply turned his back to me and refused to speak anymore. Not only did he make it very clear that he did not want Jeanette to marry me, but—in his mind —I was the worst possible candidate for his beloved daughter. I'm pretty certain he carried that opinion of me for the first several years of our marriage. Sometime later, he confessed to me these lingering doubts. He even asked me to forgive him! Jeanette's mom was so different. After quietly observing Jeanette's dad give me the silent treatment, she slipped up and whispered, "Welcome to the family. Can I fix you some break-fast?" That was music to my ears.

There we were, two young people starting our lives together without hardly anything, except each other. The only thing we had was a bedroom suite that Jeanette had purchased a couple of years earlier after graduation. I had dropped out of school and was working for a local company making about one dollar an hour. Yet I was the happiest I had ever been. Oblivious to any other magical scenario than the one I conjured up in my mind, I was about to get a rude awakening. About a week after our marriage, Jeanette decided she had to have a stern talk with me about something. With a look and voice of authority that she obviously got from her father, she declared, "Now that we've settled into our apartment, I have something to talk to you about. It's very serious."

Too immature to recognize the seriousness of her tone, I jokingly responded, "Go ahead. There's no one in this apartment but the two of us."

She replied quickly and firmly, "No. It doesn't work that way. "

She led me into our small bedroom, closed the door, and said with piercing eyes staring at me, "You lied to me about your age. (I told her I was almost nineteen.) If you ever lie to me again, I will leave you."

Of course, this shocked me. I was so deeply in love with this beautiful young lady that my response was swift and predictable, "I will never lie to you again."

"Okay," she stated, "Be sure you keep your word." For Jeanette, truth was everything. "Furthermore, this September 1 you are going to re-enroll in high school and finish your diploma. You will not get anywhere without it."

My response was meant to be wise, but it was draped with sarcasm: "How am I going to go to school when I have a full-time job that requires 9-10 hour days?"

She replied with a look of all business, "Don't worry. I have already called the high school, and they are going to set you up with a special program that will not conflict with your work schedule. Furthermore, I've called the company you work for. They are putting you on second shift, so it will not conflict with your classwork."

For the first time, I got a glimpse of the woman I had married and the beautiful 66-year journey we would take. She was firm, but fair. To her, our marriage was not just a romance, but God's business, therefore her business.

Caught up in that mythical moment, too grand for that cocky seventeen-year-old to really comprehend, I both laughed and revered the moment. Where would I have ended up without this gift? To this day I cannot understand why this quick marriage even took place. And even more mysterious, why would this second generation Pentecostal and devout Christian marry someone who had never darkened the door of a Pentecostal church, let alone had a salvation experience? From our August 6 wedding date forward she never stopped praying for me. To her credit, I know it was her prayers that led me to be marvelously saved and filled with the Holy Spirit only three months after we were wed.

After only a few years adjusting to married life, we accepted the call to ministry. It was never my private call. From the very beginning it was our call. She was never separated from any of my life and ministry exploits. Together we ventured through the academic world, two adoptions and the birth of our third child, military service during the Korean War, training for missionary work, pastorates, and finally, Army Chaplaincy in Vietnam. Every decision, every struggle, every new crisis, she was with me as a co-partner. We not only survived these many years of ministry and family life, but did so with much joy and success. As I surveyed the details of our journey, especially at this juncture, I vividly remembered so many heartwarming events that could have only happened to a couple whose lives were directed by the Lord. Of course, I also recalled those more fearful times. After we were married, Jeanette continued working at the telephone company. One night she left work late. A man followed her out and then chased her for nearly an hour. Although Jeanette was fortunate enough to escape untouched, the man was later arrested and charged as a rapist. Even then we understood that the Lord not only protected us individually, but jointly. He has always been the God who was for us, watching over us, and ensuring that the great plan He had for us would not be thwarted by the evil schemes of this world.

I held tightly to Jeanette's hands, not just for her comfort, but for my reassurance that this was all going to turn out alright knowing that in our many years together we had depended upon the Lord in so many situations for healing, protection, guidance, and comfort. For me, this whole process was not about a disease; it was about a woman I dearly adored. At that moment I could not think how I would ever live my life without her.

"Jeanette Crick?" My thoughts were interrupted. Finally, they called her back.

We gathered our things to join her, but were abruptly denied entrance. The technicians explained that Jeanette needed to go back alone with them so that they would get a good reading without interruptions. It would be the beginning of a four-hour series of events including basic tests with multiple inventories, reviews and comparisons of CT-scans and MRI reports from the past four years. As I watched them lead her out of the waiting room, my own thought processes pierced my heart so deeply I believed them to be mortal wounds. *Why did it take me so long to see those symptoms?* I had many excuses, all of which seemed so inexcusable. Those early signs were there, but our busy lives delayed the doctor visits.

During our last few years at the Seminary and Chaplains Commission, we were overwhelmed with many projects and events, most of which we celebrated with joy. But these requirements pushed Jeanette and me to the point of exhaustion. I had just retired from our denomination's Chaplains Commission where I had been director for thirty-two years. Prior to that, I was fully absorbed in the building of a million-dollar Chaplaincy and Care Center in Romania. I was so busy—too busy to notice or to take serious these early signs. They came with a great cost: I was doing good things at the expense of neglecting the most precious gift of my life. Much later, when I finally confessed my feelings of guilt to Jeanette, she assured me by patting my hands and saying, "You did all you could do and more than most."

Yet, on that most unforgettable day in the waiting room I could not disconnect from that deep-seated accusation: *Why? Why did I not do more, sooner?* My mind went to those events of missing car keys, forgetting her favorite niece's name, and struggling to balance our checkbook. Then there were the more obvious events. Two years earlier I was suddenly awakened at about four in the morning. Jeanette had fallen down a flight of steps trying to find the bathroom. Even though she had claimed she was okay, I now anguished over not insisting she go to the ER. I wondered if that could have been the beginning of what our family doctor later described as "mini-strokes." My heart was pierced again by the invasion of "why?" Why did I not override Jeanette and the doctor's opinions and rush her immediately to the emergency room? Maybe she would have been referred to a specialist that very night.

Instead I relied on the advice of well-intentioned friends who were also our physicians. We travelled together and went on missionary trips together. We hung out together and worshipped together. So when I first began to notice signs of memory loss, difficulties completing daily activities, and other unusual behaviors, I reported this to our friends in the medical profession. I even made an appointment with one and described her growing difficulties at work and at home. The general response was that she was growing older. When things got serious enough for me to go against my family doctor's recommendations, I consulted with another physician who referred her, on my insistence, to the Wesley Woods Memory Disorders Clinic. Located at the Emory University Hospital, Wesley Woods was one of three top treatment and research facilities in the nation

34

and they were known for their long-term efforts to find better treatment plans and possibly a cure for Alzheimer's. I also had a personal attachment to the Clinic. In 1972, I was sent there to complete my doctoral and clinical studies in preparation for Clinical Pastoral Education Supervision.[9] I supervised students doing clinical pastoral work with patients and families connected to the Center. I had a firsthand look at Alzheimer's disease. Who would believe that our journey would take us right back to these grounds? Now, as patient and spouse, we waited to hear those formidable words, "Your wife has Alzheimer's."

Of course, Jeanette and I had lived through many crises and near death experiences. Maybe I too easily believed that God would just handle all of these evolving issues. It had been both our experience and our belief that we served a Lord who declared, "By His stripes, we are healed" (Isaiah 53:5). As I scanned through the evidences of our lives, rehearsing moments of miraculous interventions, my mind drifted to 1968 at Fort Benning, GA, where Jeanette lay in a coma for three days. Our young military surgical team told me that they did not have a clue as to what was causing her high fever and organs to shut down. Her condition was so severe that the Catholic priest provided by the military asked permission to give her the sacrament of "Last Rites." Only by a miracle of circumstances did one of the doctors consult with an older specialist who advised, as a last effort

---

9 Clinical Pastoral Education is part of the educational process chaplains must complete in order to become Board Certified. This training is both theological and practical. It provides direct supervision for students as they learn how to minister to individuals and families in crisis. CPE Supervisors must undergo many additional hours of training. For more information visit the ACPE website at www.acpe.edu.

at saving her life, to do exploratory surgery. The entire Christian community of Fort Benning was praying for her. During surgery they discovered that her fallopian tube had burst from a tubal pregnancy, and she was suffering from infection spreading throughout her system. When she awakened from her surgery, several doctors were standing at the foot of her bed. The lead surgeon shook his head. When Jeanette asked why he was doing so, he stated, "We did not save you; it was the handiwork of our Savior." Facing this new crisis of Alzheimer's, I found myself again in deep conversation with the Lord. My prayers were as basic as it gets in a crisis of this magnitude: *You saved her back then, and have preserved her all these years for life with her family and ministries around the world. Why not again?*

I was suddenly pulled out of my prayer to the sound of Jonne, my daughter, saying, "Dad, you got to come and help us. Mom is not cooperating with the technicians who are administering the Alzheimer inventories."

I hurried to her room.

Overcome with fatigue, I couldn't help but have contemptuous thoughts about that place. Those same technicians who wouldn't allow us to remain with her were now begging us to come and assist them. When I got back to the testing room, Jeanette was sitting on the floor, exhausted from all the inventories and frustrated with those administering the tests. Like a stubborn child, she had finally had enough. The inventories, which should have taken only an hour, had taken more than two hours at this point. We had already travelled many miles to get to the Clinic, waited two hours for them to see her, and now completely worn out, Jeanette pleaded with me, "Bob, please, if you care one ounce for me, take me home!"

When I asked her what was wrong, she reported, "I am tired of them treating me like a child. Asking me silly questions like, 'Where were you born? What is your social security number? Can you remember the name of the place I told you about earlier?'"

In her pre-Alzheimer state, Jeanette assisted some of our seminary professors in administering and evaluating exams. This experience was so far removed from *that* Jeanette. The "adult Jeanette" had been momentarily pushed aside in this new "Alzheimer's state" for that of a stubborn child.

Rightly so, Jeanette, the stubborn child, was done. After a long day of travelling and waiting, she was already tired and frustrated. To add to her growing frustration, the clinic was going through its own transition. They had just moved into a new office and were operating in a bit of confusion. Due to the many delays and interruptions (including several missing medical assistants, clients who got loose and were running down the clinic halls, and the psychiatrist leaving to attend to these issues), Jeanette had very little left to offer. And her exhaustion led to a greater experience of confusion and stress which was evident from beginning to end.

We all learned many things during her first extensive evaluation. I learned how both family and clinic can be unprepared for such a long and arduous assessment. These inventories should have been rescheduled. What we thought would be a simple matter of a well-processed and interpreted Alzheimer's inventory did not happen so simply. The whole process, like the disease, was complex. I knew then that I had to get ahead of the process.

The best thing that happened during this visit was the doctor's careful analysis of Jeanette's MRI. This appeared to be his greatest skill. With all the pragmatism of a clinician and very little warmth, he gave us the news. The news I dreaded. The news I feared. The news that I deep down already knew. "Dr. Crick, your wife has all the signs of Alzheimer's disease." There it is, the moment. The moment that awakened me to a new reality in our lives. A reality that had been with us for some time. A reality we refused to acknowledge. What can I say? To hear the words that your wife of so many years, a companion and co-partner, the mother of your children and the grandmother of your five grand kids, is now diagnosed with Alzheimer's…it is silence in slow motion. Forget about how much you think you know about this disease; you know nothing until you hear those words, *Jeanette is in the early to middle stages of Alzheimer's.* It awakens you. It demands your attention. It forces you into an elongated moment. This moment—though only a moment—lingered for what seemed like a lifetime. Our lifetime. I fought in that moment through shock and despair. I fought for *our moment,* our lifetime of moments. He didn't stop for my moment. She didn't seem to notice the moment but it was there. Engulfing us, engulfing me, and permeating the very depth of my soul—for a moment. But I'm a clinician, a professional. I had to face up to the fact that Jeanette had a terminal disease that would eventually take her life. So I forced myself out of that moment—still barely able to keep up with the moment—to listen attentively to his thorough interpretation of the MRI. He explained that the disease had already done its initial damage around the outer edges of the brain cortex. It was well on its way to its destructive finality. He advised we needed to have a plan for her care.

Alzheimer's. Plan. Finality. My Jeanette? Things moved too rapidly to try to catch up.

I quickly recognized I had to find a way to personalize a plan for Jeanette, and not succumb to a pre-arranged, one-size-fits-all packet. She deserved a plan that fit who she was as a person and client, one that took into consideration not only what these specialists valued, but what she and "we" valued—her unique story, ethics, and spiritual needs.

I found myself asking, "Where is God in this?" Only, this time, there were no immediate, forthcoming answers.

Every once in a while, I would break eye contact to check on Jeanette. I wondered how she was holding up. Was the news crushing her like it was crushing me? The weight too much to bear, I found myself asking that question I often posed to my Clinical Pastoral Education students, "Where is God in this?" Only, this time, there were no immediate, forthcoming answers. I felt utterly alone in our news. Fortunately, Jeanette was too tired to even listen to his extensive, in-depth analysis and had lost focus very early.

When the doctor stopped speaking, the next wave of moments hit. The after-shock moments. The questions with no answers moment. What do we do now? Who do we get to assist us in this battle? Where is our God? How do we respond to all the practical issues like security, a treatment plan, and nutrition? How do we even begin this journey? And the most painful, why my Jeanette? Did God forget who she was and the kind of godly woman she had always been? She served this world, His people, with diligence, kindness, wisdom, and power. With no answers in sight, I pulled myself out of that despairing chair and prepared for the long trip home.

No one spoke for most of the ride home. We couldn't if we tried. The silence was just too loud to speak over. And so dense we would have been swallowed up by it if we opened our mouths. I wanted it to be a "be still and know that I am God" moment, but it was a "deep calling unto deep" moment. My soul was overwhelmed, beaten down by the weight of the whitewater rapids, the breaking surf, the thundering breakers. It was too much. It was a crushing like waves that returned and swelled almost rhythmically upon my heart. Never relenting. I was engulfed by intrusive thoughts. Her impending death sentence...no record of anyone being healed of Alzheimer's...the awareness that we had begun a journey that there was no turning back from. Like the psalmist in Psalm 42, I sensed a deep despair dragging me under. Then, out of the quiet, an unlikely standard was raised on our behalf. A breaking of the weighted silence.

It was Jeanette who finally broke through the silence. None of us could have handled the news like her. Rather reflectively, in her own altered state, she determined, as she sat beside me in the car, "Bob, I don't like that place. And, I don't think *they* know what they are doing."

Her pragmatic response, so oblivious to her own plight, broke the ice for Jonne and me. I don't know whether it was the oddity of her evaluation or her pragmatism in our moment of crisis, but we broke out into laughter. This is the God we serve. The God who binds us to His joy when the sirens of crisis call out to us to jump ship. Psalm 42:8 declares, "Then [after the experience of crushing], God promises to love me all day, sing songs all through the night! My life [your life and her life] is God's prayer!" (The Message, commentary added). I was assured in that moment that though we would surely get tossed and turned, He wouldn't let Jeanette or me go under. For He is indeed the lifter of our heads and the standard that protects us from the floods of this world. While devastation still touches us, He does not leave us without defense. He is a God of covenant, bound to us relationally, lovingly. Just as I am bound relationally and lovingly to Jeanette. It is a bond too wonderful to deny and too wonderful to fail.

Chapter 2

Until Death Do Us Part: More than a Vow, a Covenant

"You have captivated my heart, my sister, my bride."
—*Song of Solomon 4:9 (ESV)*

The realities of such a harsh awakening can momentarily cause one to experience a measure of dissonance or confusion. That internal vision becomes blurred—even doubled. So instead of a singular path through a well-manicured park, a person sees multiple paths through a dark and impenetrable forest. The journey itself is too big, too daunting, and too fearful. It paralyzes even the best of us, momentarily. Maybe that is a gift, for paralysis forces us to be still and face truths that we desperately want to run from. It forces us to carefully examine where our commitments truly lie and where they must be transferred. A sacrifice we were unwittingly willing to make as we sought to navigate through the daunting news of her diagnosis and then look ahead to find an entry point into a new and unknown journey for our family.

I wish I could say that the movement from our awakening to commitment to strategy was seamless—that we excelled even our own expectations, never losing our footing or succumbing to moments of despair and regret. But that simply wasn't our story. Our story doesn't easily move from scene to scene seamlessly, as you will surely note. Rather, awakened to the fact that we were in the midst of a story already in full motion, we were simply trying to catch up with the author and finisher of that story. While seemingly counter-productive, our moment of paralysis became the necessary force which propelled us forward. It was our moment of regrouping and self-examination. First we re-examined our commitments and more fully defined our relationship based on the unbreakable, biblical truths of covenantal love. Then we looked back, examined our story and how we ended up where we were, looked forward to that inevitable end, and from those negotiations mapped out—the best we could—a strategy that would allow us to remain faithful to the story, the journey we were called to live.

While the first announcement of Jeanette's Alzheimer's disease may have temporarily dazed and confused us—even partially paralyzed us—we very quickly did what we had always done: we sought the Lord with our family and closest friends. As we prayed together, we asked the Lord for guidance on how we would—could—negotiate this process. Almost immediately it became *our shared* journey. After twenty years of military chaplaincy, the life and language of the sojourner was rather common to our experiences. Serving during Vietnam, our transience was of biblical caliber—moving from station to station all over this world. The presence of the Lord was our mobile and immanent stay. Like clockwork Jeanette would call a "conference" to inform the kids that I had been transferred yet again.

Then a long negotiation process would begin. *What does this mean for our family and for each of us?* With the news of her diagnosis, Jeanette again brought us back to the table. While I don't remember her exact words, in my heart I'm certain she was reassuring us, even declaring over us, this promise: "We are *moving*, again, but don't worry the Lord will go ahead of us, and He will prepare the way."

In spite of her assurances, it was our nature to question, "What will this new journey mean for us?"

Many families face similar negotiation processes every day with news of sickness and disease, loss of jobs, tragic circumstances within the community, and death. When such an event or change takes place, these families—our families—are faced with the challenge to revisit their commitments. For us, this meant we must decide whether our past and present circumstances, our spiritual and emotional well-being, and the extent of our willingness to be selfishly-selfless would lead us to a contractual or covenantal commitment with one another. It was not our nature to contract our loyalties. As the people of God, our commitment had to be founded in the relational nature of a covenant. Therefore, as covenant people, there was only one reasonable response. Jeanette's final journey would call us to covenant with one another and with her. There was no demanding of our loyalties; rather, an invitation to be fully engaged in the process. And we were determined to oblige if it allowed us to remain with her as long as we were able. For this is the language of love. And as we discovered, this covenantal love-language is universal transcending even the land and language of Alzheimer's.

Differentiating between contractual and covenantal love was very important to us. That difference established how we would love her and bind ourselves to her until the bitter end. Thus, contracts can be described as something necessary but temporary. We make contracts in buying a new automobile, planning a vacation, or some other short-lived agreement that, once the promise is fulfilled, the agreements are completed. Contracts are the way we describe many of our short-term experiences that are necessary but not permanent. Jeanette and I had lived through many experiences which we would label as contractual. Being in military chaplaincy, there were many short-term assignments, some as short as a month and others as long as several years. We made friends in these short assignments and had some remarkable experiences in new and interesting cultures. But in most of these assignments, long-term relationships were rarely formed.

Covenants, on the other hand, are different both in content and policy. A covenant by its nature is everlasting because it is God-ordained. It is not established upon mutual self-interest. In fact, what makes a covenant so much more powerful than a contract is that a contract is an exchange of goods and promises for a limited period of time, but a covenant is an exchange of persons established by an oath which creates an everlasting *kinship.*[10] Two become one. A blood covenant is offered. This is why the groom can refer to the Shulamite as his sister, his bride (Song of Sol. 4:9-12, 5:1-2). Her

---

10   Scott Hahn, "Contract versus Covenant," Outlook, Worldview Publications, February 2002. Web 15 August 2015. http://www.worldviewpublications.org/outlook/archive/main.php?EDITION=043.

sistership (figuratively) makes her a blood relative—an unbreakable bond; her *brideship* makes her the chosen recipient of his oath to care for, protect, and love "until death do them part." The oath is the central piece of this commitment. According to David Foster,[11] to make an oath is to "[draw down] the presence of God... for help... so that we can do whatever it is that we are pledging to do." This is how Jeanette and I covenanted with each other all of our years together. Even as we sat painstakingly evaluating our negotiations, I sensed the Lord being drawn into the moment, strengthening us— me—to carry out my oath of love, commitment, compassion, and care. Only as the journey moved forward did I really understand that this oath would look more and more like our Lord's commitments to us. There would be no balance or reciprocity. She can't offer a mutual love. She was simply my beloved—the object and desire of my care. This deepened covenant, dependent on the presence of God, is about her needs and my willingness to meeting her needs. So I covenanted with her, again, in my heart—not because she was the lesser of the two, but because she was the one most prized.

> *I covenanted with her, again, in my heart — not because she was the lesser of the two, but because she was the one most prized.*

Our marriage was already based on a loving, God-centered, self-less kinship that developed and grew over our lifetime with each

---

11   David K. Foster, "Covenant: The Heart of the Marriage Mystery," Focus on the Family, n.d. Web. 15 August 2015, http://www.focusonthefamily.com/marriage/gods-design-for-marriage/marriage-gods-idea/covenant-the-heart-of-the-marriage-mystery.

other. But in our negotiations, the covenant expanded. Not because she asked or even demanded it of me; rather, I discovered anew that my most prized treasure and invaluable family heirloom was Jeanette. Her life and her legacy was too costly to deny, too precious to be stored away. No, in my life—like God is with us—she must be given a place of prominence. Don't mistake my evaluation as a romanticized version of the truth. It is a bloody covenant initiated for the sole benefit of the other person.[12] That is, no matter if she can hold up her end of the bargain— which she can't—I *must* hold up mine.[13] I, more than I wanted to, got it. This kind of a covenant is unconditional and permanent.[14] But it was the only real gift I could give her now.

> *This kind of a covenant is unconditional and permanent. But it was the only real gift I could give her now.*

We did not come by this love accidentally, but providentially. Even as a young couple the Lord was already shaping these concepts into the very fabric of our relationship. We were determined that our life together would be orchestrated by the Lord. I don't want

12 Gary Chapman, "Marriage: Covenant or Contract?" Lifeway, 3 January 2014. Web. 8 August 2015, http://www.lifeway.com/Article/HomeLife-Marriage-Covenant-or-Contract.

13 Herman Ridderbos, "The Epistle of Paul to the Churches of Galatia," (Grand Rapids: Eerdmans, 1953: 130-31), quoted on Bible Research, Covenant, n.d. Web. 8 August 2015, http://www.bible-researcher.com/covenant.html.

14 Gary Chapman, "Marriage: Covenant or Contract?" Lifeway, 3 January 2014. Web. 8 August 2015, http://www.lifeway.com/Article/HomeLife-Marriage-Covenant-or-Contract.

to overstate this point. We had all the human experiences of any young family, but, because of our unique family histories, we both were looking for something deeper than just a relationship. We sought, even hungered for, something far more stable and more fulfilling than our previous experiences in our large families of origin. Commitments that were born out of more than just duty. Commitments born out of love and respect and selflessness. Jeanette displays this desire best in a letter she wrote to me while I was in Vietnam:

October 22, 1966

Dearest Bob,

Some in the family said that if they weren't married, they would never get married. I told them they must be miserable people with their companion, but that does not apply to me. In truth the years of my marriage have been the happiest I've ever had. There were so many of us at home [growing up] that I was ready to be free from my parents. Of course, it is only after you grow up that you begin to appreciate your parents. I hope we remember that while ours kids are growing up. The day I met you and that day we were married I became only yours. Then, I really knew what it was to have someone to love me. It hasn't been peachy these 18 years. It's funny how afterwards the only things you really remember are the peachy things, those wonderful memories of your romance. Oh, one thing is for sure, I'm a happy companion of yours. I would rather have you with me and have nothing, not even any money…

Love you with all my heart and soul,

Jeanette

Our story is certainly not a new one. It is watermarked by the countless stories of God's people, most notably the Israelites. Like us, the Israelites were fragmented and nomadic. They roamed the desert lands with a strange, almost mysterious sense of wanting something more permanent. That Old Testament scene parallels what Jeanette and I were seeking in our relationship. In our early years, we too were tired of being fragmented, without a permanent home, and without a permanent leader. We were mere nomads in those days, drifting with an insatiable hunger for a permanent home and a permanent spiritual relationship. We found those things in a holy God who declared to us in Leviticus 26:12, "I will be your God and you will be my people." This covenant-keeping Abba-God never relented in his promise of being our faithful and everlasting God. It was our Truth, not philosophically or idealistically, but intimately and experientially.

In those early years, we began talking about finding ways to deepen our relationship with each other and with the Lord. Too "green" yet to understand the depth of a covenantal marriage, the Lord was leading us toward a marriage bond only understood through spiritual eyes. It was a bond that tied us together through geographical distances, near death experiences, grief and loss, and major life transitions. It was a bond so powerful that it could only have been created by an omnipotent, Creator God. Our not-yet realized, covenantal marriage was a God-design. This kind of marriage calls on us to be generous in our gift of self and resources. In its origins is the image of a great God who extends to a vulnerable and finite being his oath of care and protection. By its very nature, it is a one-party guarantee.[15] The "lesser" partner cannot possibly offer anything of significance in return, except faith in the oath. This is how we saw one another. A deep sense of wanting to care for the other through all things, life.

By the time our family and ministries were well established, the word covenant had become almost a household word for us maneuvering through life's journey. No longer limited to Jeanette and me, it represented how we committed ourselves to one another and our children. From the beginning it was our desire to have children, but we couldn't. So, after thirteen years of waiting, we adopted David, our oldest child. Not wanting him to be alone, we decided to adopt again. However, this adoption did not come so easily. Stationed in Germany, we sought help through a German adoption agency. At first we ran into a hardheaded German bureaucrat who did not want one of *his German kids* to be raised in an American home. Refusing to give up, we went over his head and found a wonderful

---

15   Gary Chapman, "Marriage: Covenant or Contract?" Lifeway, 3 January 2014. Web. 8 August 2015, http://www.lifeway.com/Article/HomeLife-Marriage-Covenant-or-Contract; Herman Ridderbos, "The Epistle of Paul to the Churches of Galatia," (Grand Rapids: Eerdmans, 1953: 130-31), quoted on Bible Research, Covenant, n.d. Web. 8 August 2015, http://www.bible-researcher.com/covenant.html.

German social worker who led us through all the "red tape." Once approved, we chose a beautiful, German baby girl, Jonne Lynn, as our one and only choice. She was to be placed in our home once she reached three months old. However, miraculously, in the midst of the adoption, Jeanette became pregnant with our youngest child, Dale. The social worker was unsure about how all this would work out and questioned our commitment to Jonne. But Jeanette and I could not get away from two powerful "covenant" images. First, we couldn't shake the image of that little baby girl who was waiting for us, her new mom and dad, to come and get her. Whether she was cognizant of it or not, we bonded—covenanted—from the moment we saw her, chose her, held her. She was ours, and we were hers. Second, we knew this bond was the result of prayer. In fact, one of the Catholic nuns at the orphanage declared on our first visit, "This baby is my special angel, and I am so happy the Lord sent to me a pastoral family to raise her up in a Christian home. That is an answer to my prayers." As we held Jonne for the first time, this dear Sister made us promise that we would not change our minds regardless of the circumstances.

Reminded of that beautiful covenant so many years earlier, as a couple and as a family, we renewed our covenantal vows to one another—not so much with words, but in Spirit—to not change our minds about one another regardless of the circumstances. For me, our covenant was never more central to my dealings with her. Maybe it was even more in line with our biblical model. As I watched her come to terms with a disease that would make her so terribly vulnerable, I could understand better why God would enter into an oath that is one-sided. It comes from a realization of one's love and personal commitment to live out that love in real and necessary ways. It is that moment when a covenant can no longer be philosophical, but fully realized in our practical commitments and willingness to rearrange all of our lives to accommodate the need of this one person, the object of my attention, the love of my life. It is unbreakable, non-returnable. The Divine covenant, therefore, inherently implies that whether we believe God to never again send a world-wide flood or not, He won't because he vowed to us He wouldn't. Whether Sarai believed Abram would be the father of many, he would because God vowed he would. Likewise, at that moment, I became keenly aware that it didn't matter who she

As I watched her come to terms with a disease that would make her so terribly vulnerable, I could understand better why God would enter into an oath that is one-sided.

believed me to be or not to be, the responsibility of fulfilling the covenant was on me. And I was determined to do so until death do us part.

Chapter 3

Creating Our Commandments of Care: Negotiating the Non-negotiables

"Fix these words of mine in your hearts and minds;
tie them as symbols on your hands and bind them on your foreheads."
—*Deuteronomy 11:18 (NIV)*

I f you have any sense at all, you had better start now getting your house in order." Those were the doctor's words which took captive my thoughts in the coming days—even though our initial moments were given to family and covenant renewal. The urgency of his words told us life would never be the same. This would be a journey with devastating consequences. So we did not delay. Within a week after Jeanette's diagnosis, we had the family in for a sobering discussion of the process that awaited us. In our conversations, it became painfully clear that we should have started much earlier. Those daunting questions from the waiting room resurfaced; only, this time I wasn't alone. They besieged *all* of our hearts... *Why did we fail to see the early signs? Why did we let doctors convince us her problems were just aging? Why didn't we rearrange our busy schedules sooner to be with her longer and more significantly? Why?* Guilt. Regret. The other captors in my head. In all of our heads. Except, these captors were insistent on their dominant place in the discussions. There were no negotiations, no hope of release from our guilt and regret. They were our most vicious captors. Knowing we were fully unprepared to defeat them, we focused our energies on those issues we believed we were better prepared to negotiate— getting our house in order.

Our strategy was simple, but demanded of us great personal investment. We began by asking ourselves an important question, *"Have we been here before?"* As painful as it was to grasp her dreaded diagnosis, we were certain we could take on this fight as we had taken on every traumatic experience in our lives: together. This would be no different. So, we committed to meet together regularly. These meetings were our strategy meetings. We sought answers in the rehearsing of our story and God's faithfulness weaved in and through all parts of it. Nothing was untouched by His hand. These stories gave us hope and returned strength to us as we were reminded of who we were and to whom we belonged. Therefore, we bound them to us as if commands handed down to us by God himself. We bound every truth to our hearts and every image of a merciful God to our minds. We carried our stories to and from the negotiating tables. And always kept them in plain sight.

The practice of binding and rehearsing our story was a most powerful tool. It led us toward a deepened discovery of our true identity and was the means by which we confronted and cleared up our distorted identities. As a family, *our story* was the process by which we reclaimed our identities, put away false and distorted identities, and formed our deepest relationships. We were, in a sense, defining who we would be and the ethical practices we would cling to as we negotiated this next painful journey. Of course, in this early stage of her Alzheimer's, Jeanette was in on every discussion. She always let us know her feelings and desires even though at times she seemed confused and exhausted. A couple years into the process, however, she drifted into a more subdued state: no longer a leader, but a follower.

Every time we gathered, we recounted our family stories. It was our practice, our most vital negotiating strategy. Those stories were our anchors as we discussed this new chapter of our lives, with its devastating possibilities. They reminded us that God has never left us or forsaken us in any crisis or celebration. For He is not in the business of leaving His beloved people to journey alone. We had to make those truths foundational for the journey. To have ventured out without them would have been like walking through the wilderness with an empty knapsack. The results would be devastating. So I encouraged everyone to share a story that illustrated the Lord's intervention during a time of crisis. Jeanette readily shared. She told us of the time when her Dad, a coal miner in Kettle Island, KY, had nearly been killed during a mine explosion. She testified to the Lord's faithfulness through many sicknesses and surgeries, one of which almost took her life. I, too, could testify about *Jehovah-Rapha*, the God who heals. Several years into our marriage I was diagnosed with a liver infection so serious that the doctors believed I was going die. Yet God faithfully intervened and rescued me from potential death. These stories were not just scrapbook memories for our entertainment. They drew into the present an enduring faith that would ultimately sustain us deep into our imminent wilderness experience. A faith steeped in the difficult questions and solidified in those both answered and unanswered.

The doctrine of healing, the heart of those difficult questions, has always been a core belief in our faith system, taught almost as a part of our DNA and practiced with our kids and grandkids. In fact, it was my grandson who raised the question of Jeanette being healed. You see, these miracle stories drew into the present those difficult questions we could not yet answer, such as, should we be asking the Lord to heal Jeanette? It wasn't a question as to whether we believed God was able; we believed and have seen the power of God to accomplish what, in our minds, is impossible. The answer we were most interested in was whether He would choose to heal her this time, although the answer was already being called forth from my heart. I knew. I knew that even this harsh reality wasn't the merciless withholding of compassionate care from our Lord. It was absolutely in line with God's faithfulness and goodness. Though it didn't seem to make sense, this truth was freeing. Knowing, above anything else, that God was still in control relinquished me from my need to be sovereign and allowed God to do what He does best: write our stories from the end to the beginning. He doesn't forget us or trivialize our pain. He is invested in our lives, an ever-present help and invested participant in our stories.

Over the years, the Lord has expanded my understanding of healing. It is not an issue of yes or no, like a teenager asking to borrow the car. Healing is much more expansive. It comes to us in so many ways, even in death, physically or metaphorically. Healing is a truth permeating both Old and New Testament in passages like Isaiah 53:5 (NKJV), "By His stripes we are healed," and James 5:16 (KJV), "The prayer of faith shall save the sick, and the Lord shall raise him up." These aren't just lofty words in an ancient book. These are truths fully realized in the life of my own story. I should have died from that liver infection never leaving the hospital alive. But, after being prayed for and anointed with oil by our church, the life-threatening infection left. To the amazement of my doctors, I walked out of that hospital alive and well! And so, at our negotiating table, we both celebrated *Jehovah-Rapha* and agonized over the possibility that the Lord may not choose this course with Jeanette. In fact, He was already releasing me from the need to pray for healing, that something greater was written into this journey than healing.

Thankfully, God's faithfulness is not limited to the arena of healing. He has shown Himself over and over to be my protector, too. On several occasions, during my year with the 173 Airborne Brigade in Vietnam, Jeanette wrote me letters declaring the Spirit of the Lord had interrupted a church service to intercede for me and my unit on a specific date and time. In one specific instance in January of 1967, Jeanette felt led to ask the congregation to stop the service and pray for me and my Army unit. The pastor readily did so. In my return letters, I shared with her that their prayers were being lifted up at the exact time when my unit was facing imminent dangers. She had no idea that we were on a special mission in the Iron Triangle of Vietnam. I was with a small unit doing a search and destroy mission. As far I can remember, I was dangerously exposed to intense gun fire and grenade explosions. At one point, a grenade landed at my feet. By the grace of God and the obedience of that little church, it did not explode. That is the faithfulness of God! Beyond time zones and geographical barriers, He remains faithful to His people. It is as John Newton rightly declared in his famous hymn, "Amazing Grace"[16]: "through many dangers, toils and snares, I have already come; Tis [His faithful] grace that brought me safe thus far and grace will lead me home." I knew it was the hand of God, as well as Jeanette and the Church's prayers that saved me from harm and possible death. I later received the Award of the Bronze Star Medal for Heroism. Along with the award, I received a letter commending me for my actions on that day in the jungle.[17]

---

16 "His faithful" added for emphasis.

17 "Award of the Bronze Star Medal For Heroism" (At top) "TO: Chaplain (CPT) Robert D. Crick, date of action, 24 January 1967, Republic of Vietnam, Reason: "For heroism in connection with military operations against a hostile force: Chaplain Crick distinguished himself by exceptionally valorous actions on 24 January, 1967 in the Republic of Vietnam. On this day, Chaplain Crick was accompanying Bravo Company of the 1st Battalion (Airborne), 503 Infantry which was engaged on a search and destroy mission. During the operation the company flushed VC unit into the open. Chaplain Crick, even though unarmed, accompanied the infantry in the assault on the enemy. As the assault swept over the enemy, Chaplain Crick, completely disregarding the presence of the armed VC assisted the senior medic in treating the Viet Cong wounded. His evident concern for the welfare of the wounded captives and his insistence on the respectful handling of the enemy dead reflect great credit on himself and the United States Army Corps of Chaplains. Chaplain Crick's outstanding display of aggressiveness, devotion to duty and personal bravery were in keeping with the highest traditions of the military service. Authority: By direction of the President under the provisions of Executive Order 11046."

Caught up in the power and beauty of the moment, even our kids began to recount those times when, by grace, God had intervened in their lives. When my oldest son, David, was in third grade, he slipped and fell getting off the school bus. The bus driver, unaware of what had happened, ran over his legs. We rushed David to the hospital. The tires from the bus left visible imprints on his little legs. Yet there were no broken bones. Of course, all of us could give a scientific explanation for this unusual scene, as is often our nature. But for us, this story was simply another testimony of a God who faithfully and unfailingly intervenes in a way that illustrates His blessed care for us.

These early discussions were some of the most vital and meaningful discussions for our family. They were our first order of business in negotiating our new covenant together. And as our entry point, we took time to give God the praise for having guided us through so many journeys and affirmed—regardless of the outcome —He is indeed Jehovah-Rapha, the God who still heals.

The Strategy

From my awakening of this reality, right to the end when this disease took her life on August 25, 2014, I knew that it was up to me (with our children by our side) to seek the Lord for the best process by which to take this journey with Jeanette into the *land and language of Alzheimer's*. Out of our time of seeking the Lord, reflecting on His faithfulness, and celebrating His constant care, we decided that some issues must become non-negotiable. Formed from our personal and corporate stories, we decided these non-negotiables must evolve out of *who we are* and *who she is* in Christ. And we determined that our negotiations could not, would not, lead us away from our core identity. While we certainly had moments of struggle and weakness, we refused to take up those struggles and weaknesses as our cause and our person. That was our commitment, our covenant with her and with one another. From these negotiations four primary and equally important non-negotiables arose.

First, Jeanette would not be reduced in our thoughts or statements to anything less than who she had always been. Jeanette would not be a victim, a client, or any other title which distorted who she was and would always be. She was Mom, wife, child of God, grandmother, and unique citizen of this world. She possessed special gifts that have enriched our lives and those around her. Sensing the clock was ticking, I wanted her to know how she had enriched our lives. So, I encouraged our kids to say whatever they wanted to say to her and each other, now, and to make it a habit. Even the grandkids took advantage of this practice.

When they would enter the room, Jeanette would brighten up as if something very special just took her back to better days. Their visits gave her a special reason to temporarily come back to her old home. Not hindered by diagnosis or mental capacity, they would jump onto her lap, sing songs to her, give her hugs, and all the other magical gifts that come when little ones visit their *Oma*. They would even come and sit with *Oma*, combing her hair and telling her how special she was to them. In retrospect, allowing the grandkids to be participants in her care is what we did right.

Their nearness and childlike presence was her reprieve from this daunting journey.

Little did we know that this opportunity would be short-lived. Very soon, as the disease progressed, Jeanette's loss of memories would make it more and more difficult for her to process our conversations with her. As the disease progressed, she became less and less able to know who we were in relationship to her and who she was experiencing us to be as she formed "new relationships" in her mind with all of us. We all treasured the time the Lord gave us to keep alive those precious memories and stories of our past relationships. At the same time, we were challenged to be open and willing to accept whatever our relationship would be with her—in any given moment—as the disease progressed. In this regard, we committed ourselves to be the bearers of her personhood when she could no longer bear it herself. This is that private, not publicized or commercialized, face of Alzheimer's. It is not maintained medically or otherwise. The private face is borne, borne only by those who choose to be bearers of person and faith. In some ways, my faith prepared me to do so. We bear the personhood of Christ because he is no longer physically in this world to do so, and we bear His personhood because the world around us seeks to distort it and call it something that it is not. In this manner, we are continuously calling out of this world an authentic identity of Christ. I know what it means to guard the purity and totality of who I believe Christ to be in this world. Because of that, I could do the same with Jeanette, guarding and protecting her from those who would call her by anything less than who she was.

One way we chose to do this was through story telling. Feeling a sense of duty to keep her story alive, I would recount for Jeanette the many stories I learned from her about her parents. I would spend hours recounting her whole story—her birth, early years in Kettle Island, growing up in Chattanooga, life in the military and ministry, and, of course, our story as a family. I did it because her story was too important to me to lose forever to Alzheimer's; I did it because I wasn't ready to let go of her story, our story. Rehearsing our history was not only one of the more important things we did, I believe it is another thing we did well for her and for all of us. We weren't just borrowing from a great love story. We were preserving in our hearts and minds who she was when she could no longer call it out of herself.

Of course, the second most pressing issue was still the Alzheimer's specialist's words to get our house in order, immediately. We could not have fathomed how important and prophetic his words were, but we did take him serious. While Jeanette still had some level of independent thinking, we took care of bringing all our legal matters up to date. This included new wills and trust accounts, powers of attorney, medical agreements, and all those other financial and personal matters that fall into the general category of "business." I was amazed at how long this process took. Not just days or months, but years.

The third non-negotiable we settled on was to surround ourselves with a community of people that reflects who we are. Having already established our relationship as covenantal and recognizing that Alzheimer's disease is a battle that can last for many, many years (Jeanette's battle with Alzheimer's lasted for ten years), we knew right away we needed covenant partners who understood Jeanette and saw beyond her disease to remember and to relate with her as a very real person, with an interesting and real history. We talked about who, outside our family, we should consider as those we needed and wanted with us on her journey into the *land and language of Alzheimer's*. I tried to envision these travelers with us in terms of their need or ability to either enter with us at a "contractual" or "covenantal" level. Some we envisioned as partners who would and could covenant with us. Very quickly, we identified friends and family members who would join us at that deeper, more critical level of care. These are people who had a long, significant history with Jeanette and our family. They could see the larger picture, not just her Alzheimer's disease. They knew her long, wonderful history which allowed her spiritual and social gifts to emerge in her unique person. Most importantly, they would love her equally and unconditionally on good days and bad days, days when she would try our patience and days when out of her patience the mercy of God emerged and abounded in our, sometimes, trivial efforts.

Others we would need for "temporary purposes," those who could only endure a contractual relationship. Their visits were short. They avoided the more painful issues, and some were just out of touch when it came to understanding the complexities of Alzheimer's disease and its effects upon not only Jeanette but her immediate family members. Only later did we discover how necessary it was to separate out those who fell into these two categories.

Remember, this is a journey that took us and her care partners into strange, unchartered lands and languages. Greg O'Brien,[18] in writing of his Alzheimer's disease experiences, describes it as a journey into the distant planet, Pluto. According to his and numerous other accounts, as one gets deeper and deeper into the effects of this disease, it becomes increasingly necessary to narrow your fellow travelers to those who can truly covenant with the family. This small but vital community we created understood the person and the disease, and they were willing to be both a steady foundation and a mobile tabernacle—allowing God and Jeanette to navigate our perceptions, our norms, and our need to control her reality. To those special friends, extended family members, and several in-home caregivers, I am forever grateful for their presence and imprint on her journey.

Our fourth non-negotiable arose out of discussions with immediate family members. It puts forth two initial questions of *how will* "who we are" *be reflected in the model of care we provide personally and professionally?* And, *which models would best reflect Jeanette's needs and person?* First of all, we are spirit-filled believers. Thus, those spiritual needs which were pivotal to her person and life had to be an essential component of her care. A non-negotiable. We accomplished this by reading her Bible to her when she could no longer do

---

18 Greg O'Brien, On Pluto: Inside the Mind of Alzheimer's (Brewster, MA: Codfish Press, 2014).

it herself. We prayed on her behalf when words were not available to her. We rehearsed in her presence a life-long love of her Lord, Jesus Christ. Regularly, we would sing those timeless, enduring hymns of our faith. Even as the disease progressed, she would join in remembering the song word for word, with expressions of passion in her eyes and hands lifted up, occasionally experiencing the joy of the Lord in the midst of her worship offerings. Those old Pentecostal experiences never totally left her even in her new land.

With questions of identity fully satisfied, we discussed how that would affect the models of care we would choose. It was out of these discussions and examinations of the field that we came face to face with the vast and ever changing views concerning research on the drugs, diagnosis and prognosis of those with Alzheimer's. Trying to find an answer

Trying to find an answer to these questions was like trying—at times—to hear from God. I heard a lot of "yes, no, maybe, not yet, and let's let the process unfold a little more."

to these questions was like trying—at times—to hear from God. I heard a lot of "yes, no, maybe, not yet, and let's let the process unfold a little more." In the early process, we learned by trial and error—not my method of choice. Little did we know how numerous the medical and professional care plans were for those with Alzheimer's disease. To make matters worse, the plans were often confusing and contradictory. They ranged from those that recommended none of the approved drugs to those with specific plans with specific drugs and treatment models. We learned quickly that the whole field of Alzheimer's is vast with many paths and little guidance.

Choosing (and then managing) our medical personnel was a huge undertaking also. Medical personnel treating those with this disease range from nurses, family doctors, psychiatrists, psychologists, neurologists, etc. It was no easy task finding the best medical professionals to guide her and us through this long, eight-year process. Without hesitation, if we felt we were not getting the best medical guidance, we changed doctors and clinics. Right up front, I learned that we were the best responders in developing an effective medical plan for Jeanette. Regardless of how many medical and social service specialists wanted to give her comprehensive personal treatment, their own loaded schedules did not allow such. So, out of necessity, we became zealous students in the "Art of Alzheimer's."

Thank God for the many books and other available resources. Staying informed not only gave us a sense of empowerment in the midst of an almost powerless journey, it kept us talking and moving forward in our efforts to provide excellent care. It is one of the many things that we did right for her. The literature we found provided necessary assistance in deciphering the multitude of information given. Among the most helpful were those individuals who wrote books recounting their loved one's journey with Alzheimer's disease and other similar illnesses, some lasting more than twenty years. Additionally, we consulted with several on-line sites almost daily, both in making those initial decisions and long-term decisions.[19] The collective information from these many resources gave us a starting point with which we could navigate through the abyss of care alternatives for her.

Fortunately, these resources helped us find good persons, clinics, and doctors who gave us adequate attention and care. Nevertheless, the doctors were often too busy for their own good. It didn't take me long to realize that not everyone shared in my commitments. Much of my early frustrations came as a result of the many doctors, nurses and other medical specialists who were not awakened to her *person*. That is, they couldn't see past the public face of Alzheimer's in order to see the private.[20] Immediately, I discovered that many professionals, like me, saw these individuals as clients rather than persons with a history to pass down and a present, continuous role to play in their families and communities. With the many time constraints, professionals have great difficulty taking the time to discover the individual whose own personhood has gotten lost within all the complexities of examinations, paper work, prescriptions, and appointments. The average time spent in an appointment

---

19 One online site that was particularly helpful was www.alzheimersreadingroom.com, passionately managed by Bob DeMarco. The site has hundreds of helpful articles and resources. I consulted it often in making these initial decisions and later in the long-term care for Jeanette. DeMarco's driving passion for this site and his other endeavors in this special field arose out of his own long-term care of a father with cancer and mother with Alzheimer's disease.

20 For more information about the public and private face of Alzheimer's disease, read through the preface entitled: The Public and Private Faces of Alzheimer's.

with the attending physician is somewhere between 5-10 minutes. As a result, I realized the vast difference between understanding and caring for *a client* versus *my wife*. Even the best doctors couldn't see that this was *my wife* and *my life partner* for more than sixty years.

A deep desire grew within me to humanize her in the process. It was my mission to make them understand that they were treating her, not just a disease. She was more than that. I developed a small booklet telling of Jeanette's history entitled, *The Person: Katherine Jeanette Crick*. I gave a copy of this booklet to every medical and care specialist who treated or cared for her. This booklet told of her birth and life as a child of the Great Depression; it told of her intelligence and unique skills that were noticed by teachers throughout her academic endeavors; it recounted her church ministries, marriage, family, kids and grandkids, vocational successes, and her unrelenting support of my ministry activities both in the US and other countries. The booklet was intended to alert those caring for her to not just treat the disease, but to treat Jeanette—a very unique and loving person, whose history should be celebrated, not dismissed. Of course, I got mixed reactions from doctors and other medical specialists. Some took the booklet, read it and during visits would refer to her unique history. Others, frankly, resented me for giving them this added burden, as if to say, *to me she is and will remain simply a "client."* One was honest enough to tell me he simply did not have time to form a "personal" relationship with his many clients. He even took time to tell me about the "good old days" when a physician knew his/her patients and even occasionally shared social events with them.

In spite of these hurdles, the Lord did provide several excellent care givers. However, we discovered that the best care was that managed by family and select friends who were clearly operating at the "covenant level." One of the kids stated early in our negotiations, *"Dad, please, let's not let someone else be responsible for Mom's care. We need to do it even if it requires rearranging our entire lives."*

Little did we know that this promise would stretch us almost to the point of breaking. I'm not suggesting we did it alone. We needed the extra help from in-home aides, nurses, and many others. Fortunately, we found professional helpers who provided compassionate care and communicated personal worth, but nothing will even come close to the type of care a dedicated family can provide. We were her primary care-givers. We were determined to not give away the privilege of caring for her even at great personal cost. This was the answer to our fourth non-negotiable.

Even with the best made plans, life gives us some unexpected bumps in the road.

We loved Jeanette. And although it felt at times like we were playing darts with our eyes shut rarely hitting our mark, we determined from the very beginning that this would be the most important decision-making process we would ever encounter. We wanted our commitment to be built on a foundation of integrity, honesty and trust. We wanted a plan, a strategy, which was solid both personally and professionally, with checks and balances that would enable us to stay the course to the very end, and to do so with deep faith in the Lord's guidance. Of course, even with the best made plans, life gives us some unexpected bumps in the road. Still we travailed clinging to those Truths which sustained the whole of our story. Truths like John 14:27: "Do not let your hearts be troubled and do not be afraid." Why? Because He doesn't leave us the fleeting peace this world markets for novel consumers. He gives us His peace, and like all things that belong to God, His peace is marked by its ability to endure and sustain its recipients. And He did, over and over, attentive to our brokenness and need of his constant presence. His Truth led the psalmist to conclude that there is no place we can go from His Spirit nor flee from His presence (Psalm 139). Whether in heaven, hell, or the Land of Alzheimer's, even there He will remain with us, guiding us even in the darkest of times. And, His Truth—written on our hearts and bound to our soul—sustains us, though our world gives way and our greatest strategies crumble before us.

There were many tears, doubts, and fears along the way. Some of our family, initially, felt detached, in that they lived some distance from our home in Cumming, Georgia. They complained that they were not always well informed with the twists and turns that these negotiations took. But, as we got further and deeper into the process of her journey, those small issues began to fade among the larger issues of life and death. I think we all had good intentions, but, occasionally, we reverted back to contracts and somehow let our initial covenants fade. Thankfully, when our covenant was interrupted, we had the good sense to call a conference to re-examine and to renegotiate. For the most part, we stayed the course. We did so because this disease was very personal. It was taking over the mind and body of one that we loved and so depended upon for her love and wisdom over these many years. Without any choice, she was going on her last trip into a new land and a new language, and we were invited by our love for her and conscience of faith to go with her as far as the Lord would allow. We discovered, along the way, she would go through a transformational process and so would we. The challenges of this long journey would test us at all levels: financially, spiritually, socially, and relationally. All of these changes, which we determined to be orchestrated by our Lord would be necessary, but, oh, so painful. There were times we could and would travel very closely with Jeanette into the deeper aspects of her challenging journey and times when we dropped off by the wayside only to be under conviction. Submitting in obedience to the Spirit urging us to remain faithful to our covenant, soon we would get right back into the painful process. It was a process we thought we were prepared to endure—even decided that we had been here before—only to discover this journey was one of a kind.

Over time we learned our greatest teacher and leader was the center of all our attention, Jeanette, and we were determined to be her best students. She taught us so much about ourselves and the God she (we) served. In her final role of leading us through our negotiating process, she taught us that *our task* was clear: follow her on this God-ordained Journey, be a good learner, allow the Lord to direct all journeying partners by His Word and Spirit, and expect such an important journey to be transformational. In that moment, I understood—in part—that once Jeanette's journey was complete, I must embrace these experiences and share them with others so that all of us, especially our family members, would become witnesses of His Goodness and His Faithfulness.

Chapter 4

A Light unto Our Path: Trusting God to Make Crooked Paths Straight

E ven with a good plan, we sometimes feel very lost in the process. Routinely, we brought ourselves back to the table to evaluate our progress and, at times, renegotiate our strategy. Tired, overwhelmed, and feeling like we were on anything but a well-lit path, we maintained our practice of rehearsing our story, encouraging each other to find God in the past and the present. Over time what emerged was a clear path and the assurance that God had been leading our journey long before we knew we were on it, for nothing escapes the attention of God. He always knew this would be our story. In those days, I couldn't help but cling to the Lord's promises in Jeremiah 29:11 (MSG): "I know what I'm doing. I have it all planned out—plans to take care of you, not abandon you, plans to give you the future you hope for." This passage points to a most certain assurance…He has a plan and He knows what He is doing. The peace in this knowledge is that I didn't—we didn't—have to have it all figured out. We just needed to believe that He was trustworthy, that His Word wasn't a cheap, self-help cliché with no substance. It was timelessly on time and on pace with His Kingdom's Mission. Looking back, we discovered how on pace this Jehovah-God really was.

Beginning around the year 2000, Jeanette began to sense in her Spirit a looming change. These early intuitive feelings told us that we were about to go on a journey which we had never been on before. I know now that this was God's way of preparing us for the harsh realities of Alzheimer's. This type of attentiveness to His beloved was in every way characteristic of the loving, Abba-Father whom we serve. He never forgets and never fails those who belong to Him. He is a good God who equips those He calls. We were called to this journey and most certainly equipped for it, too. These preparations were born in the heart of Jeanette.

> *I know what I'm doing. I have it all planned out—plans to take care of you, not abandon you, plans to give you the future you hope for.*

She possessed a kind of spiritual intuition that was uncanny as if she had eyes in the back of her head, especially with the kids.

When they were young, she seemed to always find them out. Every once in a while, they would sneak out to the local store thinking no one could possibly know where they were. Then, over the PA system they would hear, "Is there a Dale, David, and Jonne Crick in the store? Your mom is on the phone."

They were mystified by her omniscience. How could she possibly know where they were? With fear and trembling, they would make that long walk to the phone and then home for their reckoning. Some kids are experiential learners: they learn by doing. My kids learned by doing and doing and doing. Every time, without fail, she tracked them down and called them home. In many ways, she never stopped doing that. Always faithful to her children, she would call out to them in love and accountability drawing them back to the core of who they are in Christ and to the shelter of our home.

Call it what you want, but we knew it was the work of the Holy Spirit. As early as five to seven years prior to her diagnosis, she began having conversations about feeling something moving *toward us*. I had learned to trust her instincts as the Spirit's guidance, so we right away kept ourselves in prayer. This was before any real clues manifested, so we had no idea what was coming our way. There was no fear, just trust. We trusted the Lord would do what He had always done, walk with us and watch over us.

The Holy Spirit had used Jeanette many times in our marriage to prepare us for an upcoming transition. On two occasions, she sensed months ahead that I was going to get military orders for some special assignment. She very casually would ask if we were moving again. Knowing how the military operates, I would dismiss her question with a simple rationale: the military doesn't like to move families too quickly from an assignment. It is too costly. Sure enough, the orders would come: *Sorry for the short notice, but we need you for a special assignment. Your family will need to move quickly.* In those days, her "intuition" had become so common place that we often took it for granted, even joked about it. Until one day, the Lord showed me in a very real way that what she experienced was more than intuition, it was the Spirit of the Lord revealing and directing her on our behalf... .

Jeanette and I were experiencing probably our best military pastoral assignment at a large military installation at Bad Kreuznach, Germany. This post housed the Eighth Infantry Division. Even though I had only been serving as a chaplain for a couple of years, I was transferred to this Divisional Post to be the director of one of the largest chapel programs in Germany at that time. Long before we arrived in 1963, Jeanette and I went into a season of prayer and fasting. This program needed to experience restoration and renewal. The expectations on us were high. As a young chaplain, this is the type of assignment that could make or break your career in a hurry. But we felt that the Lord was getting ready to do something very special in our ministry. To everyone's surprise, within just a few months, our chapel attendance went from 200 to well over 500. Already, in a short period of time many had come to know the Lord. With the help of my staff, we successfully strengthened our Sunday school, Bible study groups, choirs, and counseling services. God was moving in a most powerful manner. Nearly exhausted from all the work that it took to reestablish this solid evangelical work, we planned a seven-day camping trip to England. At that time, we only had our one child, David, who was merely two years old. However, this was also the time frame in which we had arranged to adopt Jonne, our middle child from a Catholic orphanage in Worms, Germany. So needing some time away from our heavy pastoral duties and knowing that we would very soon have a new baby to attend to, we arranged for our week in England.

Everything in England went well, but two things happened that would change our life and ministry forever. First, while in England, Jeanette became extremely sick, so sick that we finally sought out an English physician for assistance. On the way to the clinic, Jeanette said, "I think I may be pregnant."

My immediate "*faith*" response was, "I don't think so. We've tried for fifteen years. Why would you be pregnant now?"

She responded, "Because the Lord told me years ago I would *birth* a child."

Affirming her only with my words and not my heart, I took her to the doctor so that we could get to the bottom of her real issue. When we got there, this older English doctor, rather humorously, put his hands on each of our shoulders and stated with a big smile, "Don't you dummies know anything about life? This young lady is pregnant! She has morning sickness."

I was equally dumbfounded and rebuked for my lack of faith. You have to understand that Jeanette and I had been trying to have a baby for years. Now after adopting our wonderful son David, and getting ready to adopt Jonne, we were pregnant? It didn't make sense; it wasn't reasonable…*my reasonable*. Fortunately, reasonableness is best decided in the heavenlies. God always has a different take on what is reasonable, for who can truly know the mind of God except that He is wholly trustworthy? Confused and elated, we decided from the start, reasonable or not, these three kids were going to be part of the Lord's master plan for our life and ministry.

On our way back from our weeklong vacation, a second life changing event occurred. While driving, Jeanette suddenly made me stop the car. Without much explanation, she stated, "The Lord just revealed to me that something has happened to Margaret."

Margaret was the fifteen-year-old daughter of our Command Chaplain and his wife. She was a solid Christian and very active in our chapel programs for teens. Our families were very close. So close that Margaret was scheduled to stay with us for two weeks following our return, while her mom and dad made a trip to Washington, DC, on military business.

Jeanette's conviction about Margaret was so strong I couldn't help but believe her. In fact, she would not finish the trip home until I pulled over to call and check on her. Hesitant, I called back to the base. Even then I was unsure how to approach the subject. *Who would I call? What would I say? My wife had a "premonition" that something bad was going to happen to Margaret? What if she was wrong? What would they think? What if she is right?* I knew what I had to do. I made the call. My assistant answered the phone. I briefly explained to him what Jeanette was feeling and asked him very generally if Margaret was okay? Dismissing our concerns, he replied, "Nothing is going on here. I spoke with Margaret a couple hours ago; I am sure she is okay."

The next day, we pulled into a snack bar near our home base, picked up a copy of the European Stars and Stripes Newspaper,[21] and there in three-inch bold print was the headline, "Chaplain's

---

21 "Chaplain's Teen Dead: Sergeant's Son Quizzed," Stars and Stripes (Europe Edition), June 10, 1963.

Teen Dead: Sergeant's Son Quizzed." We knew right then it was Margaret. Both of us wept bitterly, paralyzed by the incomprehensibility of her brutal murder. Recognizing the great task ahead of us, we allowed the hopelessness and despair of the news to grip us only for that moment. Then we did what good chaplains do every day; we prepared ourselves to give all the love and care possible to her dear parents. We didn't look for answers that day; we didn't have time for that. Instead we looked for Christ to be present and the Spirit to comfort.

The events of that bitter-sweet trip changed how I saw Jeanette's spiritual gift. It wasn't women's intuition or premonitions. It was something more powerful, more divine. It had to be the Lord at work within her spirit. This event was indicative of her deep relationship with the Lord and awareness of the Holy Spirit's inner voice. Those filled with the Holy Spirit typically experience him as that mystical, internal comforter. It is this "comforter" who extends to us spiritual power and blessings, who acts as a navigation system, giving guidance and direction through the complexities and many paths we face. If we will pay attention to those inner, intuitive feelings, we will never walk through this life blinded by the dark. For the Spirit of the Lord which resides in us is not overcome by the darkness we face. In fact, the Word of God states, "even the darkness will not be dark to [Him]; the night will shine like the day,

> *Even the darkness will not be dark to [Him]; the night will shine like the day, for darkness is as light to [God].*

for darkness is as light to [God]." (Ps 139:11-12, NIV). What this passage teaches us is that no matter how dark the impending or present darkness, God, manifested in the person of Jesus Christ, already overcame that darkness. And His Spirit which is present within us, comforts and guides us through that darkness—at times, even dispels it. What does all of that mean in practice? Because nothing is withheld from God (not our past, our present, nor our future), we could trust Him to lead us toward whatever dimly-lit darkness awaited us. So when Jeanette came to me believing the Holy Spirit revealed to her that something was coming toward us, I knew to trust her ability to sense the Lord's guidance. And I trusted the Lord to guide us.

We didn't wait for greater clarity about what was coming. Rather, we responded immediately to the Spirit's leading, spending many hours in our daily devotions and prayer talking about what was awaiting us. In more practical ways, we began to discuss the future. And due to Jeanette's insistence, we began to get our house in order. She seemed to know exactly how to navigate us through every necessary step. First, she wanted our wills reviewed by a lawyer. I didn't see the necessity to do so but obliged her insistence. Again Jeanette was the wiser of us. In doing this, we discovered how deficient those old legal documents were and revised them. Second, we took out long-term life insurance. Third, we began to clear out our basement where we had stored so many things over the years. One night we made a list of all the places in our years of marriage and ministry we had visited and those persons and places we wanted to revisit before we got too old to travel—a bucket list of sorts. We knew that both of us were getting nearer to that promised, glorious end. As we looked back over our lives and reflected on the many journeys the Lord had directed, we were overcome by the loving story He etched out in our human lives together. It was a wonderful gift to live and recount. In the seclusion of our basement, as an act of obedience and devotion, we liberally thanked God for His Word and for the ministries that helped form who we were in Him. Our journey through the past compelled us forward as we sensed a new responsibility to ready ourselves for whatever the Lord had in store, even death.

What do I mean by this? Allow me to digress and explain before recounting the trip which resulted from our bucket list. We believed in and practiced an integrated "End Time Theology." Death is inevitable, and even more so at our late ages. Yet we recognized a more expansive belief system to our eschaton: the end of this age, Christ's return, and the age to come. We weren't morbid or obsessive about the topic. To the contrary, we lived life positively and with a deep appreciation for all the good things that came our way—our love for each other, our kids, our grandkids, and those we were called to serve. However, coming out of Vietnam with many near death experiences on and off the battlefield, we developed a worldview where, for lack of a better explanation, death was an inevitable event that you either embraced or lived life in fear of. We chose the former, and in fact integrated it into our many opportunities for teaching the Word (such as Good Grief seminars), practicing pastoral care in medical centers and trauma units, as well as living out our lives as a family. We more or less factored it in as just a process of life. We had developed a faith that whether we lived or died, we were in His will and would eventually, by way of death or the Rapture, join the heavenly family for all eternity.

This belief system doesn't take away the realities of loss and grief; it merely sees how life and death can be glorious expressions of God's love for us. The truth is, our loss and grief should not lead us toward hopelessness and despair, rather to a deepened love and connectedness to a suffering Christ who sends us a Comforter to sustain us in these broken—sometimes elongated—moments.

Because we did not fear death, we were free to embrace the life we had, yet intuitive enough to begin sooner rather than later. So we planned a final trip to Europe. The entire family was in on the planning. We eagerly readied ourselves to rediscover, to touch anew, those places which were so meaningful to our family like Germany, Switzerland, and England. Of course, our planning factored in Jeanette's declining health. Jeanette was already dealing with health issues including heart problems, diabetes, and constant sinus infections. We wondered at times if the trip would even be possible. What we didn't factor was the difficulty of flying after 9/11, especially in and out of the country. We had scheduled the trip just two months after the terrible events of September 11, 2001.

When we got to the Atlanta airport to leave for England, we came face-to-face with an unbelievable crisis. The Airport had been shut down due to a security breach. Thousands were forced to leave the buildings and mass together in the surrounding streets for more than two hours. Though the incident turned out to be minor, the airport officials were taking no chances given the recent terrorist attacks. Once we were allowed in the building, we waited another three hours to get through security. Surprisingly, Jeanette held up well. We were the last to board our plane taking off nearly three hours late.

For Jeanette's comfort, I had booked the two of us first class seats, a luxury we seldom gave ourselves. I still remember to this day, as the plane took off, reaching over and taking Jeanette's hand, kissing her on the cheek, and asking her again, "Would you marry me?"

Laughing in spite of her fatigue, she responded with her usual quick wit, "Could you give me a few days to think about it?"

Although we had been married 53 years at that time, there was something very special about this trip. It was as if the Lord was allowing us that long overdue "second honeymoon." Here again I chalk it up to that inner guidance of the Holy Spirit that told us to *do whatever we needed to do for a good closure of our long life together, and to do it quickly.* Little did I know that this trip would be the last oversees trip she would ever take with me or the family. As I look back on these events, I better understand that one of these many gifts the Lord gave to me and our kids was a chance to relive some of our special times together with Jeanette. Even to this day, the kids mark this trip with their mom as the "beginning of the end." The "old Mom," who had managed our lives for so many years was fading and we knew in our hearts to grasp these fleeting moments.

Jeanette did all she could do to make the trip to England special for all of us. But she finally wore down. She spent much of our time there in her room alone reading her Bible, working on her gene-alogy charts, and listening to hymns. In the evenings, all the kids would assemble around her, telling her stories of their day's sight-seeing ventures in and around London. She listened, as she always did, with great interest and care. She was still Mom, and to her, they were still her *youngins*.

Thanksgiving Day in England was an unforgettable day. There were no thoughts of aging or lingering illnesses, just excitement about the moment. Since Thanksgiving wasn't an English holiday we were not able to find restaurants serving turkey and dressing. So we had to settle for a five-course Chinese meal as a substitute. It certainly wasn't a traditional meal, but it had all the best holiday sides of warmth, laughter, and togetherness. Our unorthodox celebration became the backdrop to our conversations about our many adventures—past and present—in Europe. When the kids were young, we had hiked in Switzerland, visited old castles in several countries, learned to ski in Austria, and so much more. Our recollection of those events were elaborate and glorious. And not 100% accurate. They moved us to laugh in spite of ourselves and in spite of a looming presence, not fully understood. I am glad that we did not know what lingered in the shadows of our meal. That shadow which leaves one haunted by the question: *What will all these special days in the future be like without Jeanette?*

Over the next few years the signs of a changing Jeanette became all too clear. She continued to do her work as the Finance Coordinator of the Chaplains Commission but not with the natural ease of past years. It took her longer, with many more hours, just to complete the very necessary tasks of the day. A person of routine, she would become greatly frustrated over her lack of focus. Every day she would work with rigor and precision at the Chaplains' Commission, read her Daily Scriptures, spend time in prayer, call her sisters and a couple select friends, read a portion of one of her Christian novels, work on her genealogy charts, and spend time with me. As time progressed, she found it more and more difficult to complete even the most rudimentary tasks. One by one they would eventually disappear. One of the last priorities to quietly go by the wayside was her daily Bible readings. Reading can be a difficult task for Alzheimer's disease patients. Because of their loss of short-term memory they can't hold on to what they read while they are reading it. The words become jumbled and the task too great to endure. Not knowing what else to do I gradually took over reading for her.

I was amazed at how her spirit refused to surrender to this disease. In spite of its devastation, Alzheimer's disease simply could not separate her from her love of God.

Through it all and almost miraculously, Jeanette's prayers remained, but not without great effort. By the latter stage of the journey, her words were often indistinguishable. In fact, during the last week before her death, she prayed many times. She prayed in short, sometimes unintelligible sentences, but always with deep, passionate feelings for the Lord, ending at times with a short outbreak of speaking in a heavenly language.[22] I was amazed

---

22 In the Pentecostal tradition, this "heavenly language" refers to speaking to God or on behalf of God in a divine language—an utterance in which the Spirit speaks and intercedes on our behalf through us in ways we cannot fully understand without the inspiration of the Holy Spirit to enlighten us.

at how her spirit refused to surrender to this disease. In spite of its devastation, Alzheimer's disease simply could not separate her from *her* love of God. As Paul reminds us in Romans chapter 8, nothing can separate us from the love of God. That includes *our love* for Him. Not trouble or hardship, not mental famine or emotional nakedness, and especially not the devastation of Alzheimer's. Nothing. More than anything else I've witnessed, her unfailing Love of God testifies to this truth. Such a love as this isn't so narrowed. It is expansive and grows with eagerness. It finds its way into the hearts and lives of many—as is true with the Love of God. I know this because the kids and I were the recipients of that Love.

Chapter 5

Nothing Can Separate Us: A Renewal of Love in Letters that Bind

"I received two wonderful letters from you today. I was so happy to get them. I read them again and again. To know that the man that I'm married to and will live with the rest of my life still has passion and desire for me. It must indeed be a miserable life for people who are married and have lost that passion and have to live together with someone they don't love and maybe with someone that doesn't love them. Your love gives me strength every day."
—*Jeanette Crick, October 24, 1966*[23]

S omewhere around 2005, Jeanette became fixated on the belief that we needed to revisit the most important experiences of our long life together. It was as if she knew *the end* was coming toward us. With her lead, we gathered the hundreds of pictures we had collected over the years, sorted them out, and put

---

23 This is an excerpt from a letter Jeanette wrote me while I was serving in Vietnam.

them into about 20 different albums. We also created for each of our children an album of their lives from birth to adulthood. The albums included all their legal documents (birth certificates & adoption papers) and pictures from their childhood, marriages, and

Revisiting that year made so much sense. It marked a major shift in our lives spiritually, vocationally, and relationally.

other memorable moments. It turned out to be a massive project that took us about two years to complete. With a sense of pride, Jeanette gave each child their own album.

Jeanette and I also dug out, at the encouragement of Dale, all the letters and reel-to-reel tapes we had shared with each other over the years, with attention to those letters written between 1966 and 1967, the year I was in Vietnam. These letters and tapes contained some of our most treasured memories and she was determined we had to revisit that season of our life through them. I have often asked myself why that year in Vietnam would be the focal point by which we began to talk about our journey coming to an end. That was such a painful year for both of us. Not only was it the first time we were separated for a long period of time, we were continuously faced with the realities of death—the unexpected loss of her father and brother, the loss of my mother, and the constant danger which surrounded me in those Vietnamese jungles.[24] Yet it was also the year that our lives took an optimal course change. It was the year the Lord deepened and strengthened our bond for each other and with our children, and it was the year He more clearly defined our specialized area of ministry. (I transitioned from regular military chaplaincy to specialized Clinical Military Chaplaincy which would later include Clinical Supervision.) In retrospect, revisiting that year made so much sense. It marked a major shift in our lives spiritually, vocationally, and relationally.

As we poured over the remains of our life together and unsuspectingly prepared for this last great journey, we were constantly reminded that a love modeled after Christ and fashioned in the heart of God could never fail. Again the Lord brought us back to Romans 8. In our limited understanding, we failed to see that the Love of God is more than just His love for us. When we house the love of God within us, we come to love like He loves—faithfully,

---

24 The 173rd Airborne (Separate) Brigade was made up of appropriately 5,000 highly trained airborne soldiers. Some 7 – 10 chaplains served this most unique unit. The Brigade was often viewed as having the flexibility to be moved from one hot spot or unexpected crisis to another. During the early part of my involvement with this unit, our mission was primarily in War Zone D, with a focus on the Viet Cong (insurgency type military units). Our unit also took part in many other major operations including Operation Junction City, where paratroopers jumped into the rice paddies at Katum in War Zone C. During the final part of my assignment, we saw extensive and bloody action in the Central Highlands near Kontum, Pleiku, and Dak To. Some of the most intense operations, many with heavy losses for US Forces, especially the 173rd Airborne Brigade, took place during the summer and fall of 1967. During the Vietnam era, the 173rd Airborne Brigade took part in 14 designated campaigns, and remained in combat longer than any other American military unit since the Revolutionary War. It earned four unit citations, had 12 Medal of Honor winners, and lost 1,601 soldiers with approximately 8,000 others wounded.

unconditionally, without end. God reminded us, as we ventured through those old letters, how steadfast His love is within those who truly love Him. We witnessed the constancy of a love not limited by circumstances, distance, or personal struggle. Now, in the aftermath of her death, I again find myself amazed at how deep our love remains within me. Indeed, not even death or the unfathomable distance of Paradise separates my heart from her love.

> *Now, in the aftermath of her death, I again find myself amazed at how deep our love remains within me. Indeed, not even death or the unfathomable distance of Paradise separates my heart from her love.*

Those old letters and reel-to-reel tapes were a record of that enduring love. Finding them in our basement was an unbelievable treasure for our whole family. It took a lot of work but *my* how we all were so happy to rediscover them. Housed in the many hours of recordings were our correspondences during Vietnam and daily devotions I had recorded for the kids during my 30 day leave prior to my tour. Around 2007 my son, David, put all the tapes on CDs for each of us. During those few years leading up to Jeanette's diagnosis, we listened to the CDs every chance we got. We listened to them to and from work, when we got together as a family, and any other opportunity that arose. We laughed in spite of ourselves; we laughed at my many formalities and Jeanette's protectiveness over me, and we cried in remembrance of our hardships and struggles. But more than anything we celebrated our youth and a time when life was so much more predictable.

Prior to going to Vietnam, I came up with the ingenious idea to record a year's worth of devotions (more than 300) for the kids on reel-to-reel tapes while separated during my tour of duty. I wanted the kids to hear my voice each day, even though as they listened I was more than 12,000 miles away in a combat zone. At the time, the kids were only five, three, and two. I desperately wanted them to feel that I was right there with them as they prepared for bed. In fact, I developed the devotions with their bedtime routines in mind. And though I wrote these to make my absence less felt for the kids, I must confess that I made them with the small hope that I too would feel less absent from them. The devotions were simple and followed the same scheme: a greeting from Dad "in a faraway place," a prayer for each of the kids and Jeanette, the scripture of the day, and a personal/family application told in the form of a bedtime story.

Jeanette, not wanting me to feel alone in the jungle, would make and send me a tape at least once a week in response to my daily devotional tapes. These tapes told of her care and activities with the kids, church life, some of her struggles with this separation, and, after she had sent the kids to bed, some personal romantic discussions of our love for each other. They and Jeanette's daily letters were my inspiration to keep the best things in my life nearest to my heart as I was experiencing the harsh realities of a dangerous combat zone. As one could imagine, these tapes were priceless to us and to me after her death.

Just as precious, but certainly more personal and intimate, were the letters Jeanette and I wrote to each other that same year. For nearly forty years, they had been left untouched, gathering dust in our basement. Yet finding them became Jeanette's personal mission. You can't imagine the joy she experienced the day we found them. Right away we determined we would read them together. The letters were deeply personal, so personal that some of their content will never be shared with anyone. They document one of the most difficult seasons of our lives. And as difficult as it was for me, it was almost unbearable for her. Rereading these letters with her reopened the guilt and powerlessness of being miles away from her, incapable of shielding her from that pain. Yet louder than my guilt was the beautiful and uplifting presence of her loving words which eased in me—to some extent—what I could not ease in her. Like so many letters written during war, they express the longing of hearts for one another, the desire to stay alive and return home, and the need to return to the blessings and presence of loved ones. Many nights we anxiously opened them one by one, like a child unwrapping a gift at Christmas. Our hearts filled with anticipation, gratitude, and joy, we poured ourselves over the contents of each letter in the privacy of our bedroom.

This time of looking back continues to be a place of comfort and satisfaction. It may have been one of the most important gifts the Lord gave to us during those last years of our journey together. Why? I can only say that to me it was the reenactment of our love in its prime. We remembered. We wept. We embraced. We celebrated. We called out the hand of God and worshiped in response.

And momentarily, we travelled back to an era that was our own personal intertwining of Renaissance and Romanticism. More fully enlightened by the documenting of our love for one another, we held tightly to what limited time we had, recognizing that even in that glorious moment that this was the Lord preparing us for whatever was coming toward us...

"When my soul is in the dumps, I rehearse everything I know of you."

—Psalm 42:6 MSG

Rehearsing All that We Knew

Night after night we pulled out of that painful era, remnants of profound love and commitment. If absence makes the heart grow fonder, then our love was in full bloom. We were incomplete without each other. Two halves desperate to be made one. In these first letters, Jeanette expressed how interdependent and intertwined our hearts were. We needed each other, unapologetically and unashamedly...

Sept. 17, 1966

Bob,

I am writing this letter with a broken heart. My Dad has now passed away. He died in the doctor's office with Virginia

95

[her oldest sister] present with him. He went so quickly. There was no chance of saving him. At his funeral, I felt I would never be happy again. He was such a wonderful dad...

If I ever needed you, today was that day. I know that if you were here, you would comfort me and take some of the hurt away. I have had two great men in my life: my dad and then you. I feel so blessed with both of you, but, as you would understand, today I am simply a "lost child." He will never again hug me. So, I have to find a way to come to grips with this loss knowing that you, where you are, need a strong wife and prayer partner. I will continue to work with these feelings, but right now please keep me in your prayers. I love you so much, and tonight I need you so badly.

Love,

Jeanette

Sept 19, 1966

Bob,

For some reason, I felt so guilty unloading on you all my pain of losing Dad. I know you understand. I did try my best to get you home to be with me, knowing you love and respect Dad. The Red Cross finally told me that, with the situation in Vietnam, they could not send you on an Emergency Leave, especially since Dad was not your dad but father-in-law.

In my grief, I believe the Lord sent me comfort last night. I dreamed about you and Dad. The Lord reminded me in the dream of when Dad visited us, just a few days before you shipped out for Vietnam. We sat together on our little porch sharing. If you will remember, he said he was so lonely without Mom [She died in 1956] …He stated that he was ready to die to join Mother, and that he would welcome death. In my dream the Lord seemed to tell me that He did exactly what Dad wanted. Now, he is with Mom for all eternity. I found for the first time some peace, and I wanted you to know that I am so much better. I still have pain losing Dad, but I still have you and the kids. This is what the Lord spoke to my heart, "Your job now is to keep praying for Bob and to take care of those little ones." Please keep giving me the assurance I need to be a good wife and a good mother. I love you so much, and I never want to lose you. To lose you would crush me forever.

Love you with all my heart and soul,

Jeanette

Sept 30, 1966

Jeanette,

I got both your letters on the same day. Honey, you and I both know that was no ordinary dream; it was right from the Lord. I have had some dreams about you, time and again, and I have come to believe that is just the Lord's way of giving us the hope we desperately need during this separation. I do not know if this helps you, but if I had been able to get an Emergency Leave to attend Dad's funeral, I would have missed a very serious operation where several of my troops were seriously wounded. [25] *I guess I am saying I was needed here, even though my heart wanted to be with you to comfort you and take care of you. At times, I feel so guilty even being in the military; it takes so many of us from our families during times like this. But, Jeanette, when I get home I will share with you stories of why the Lord has me here. Just a few days ago, one of our very best sergeants and I baptized many new converts. Had I not been here, I am not sure if they would have had the opportunity for this experience. One of them was wounded only a couple days after he gave his heart to the Lord!*

---

25   This letter was written while our 173rd Unit was engaged in "Operation Sioux City Cat Area," September and October 1966. This is where the enemy stored tons of weapons and other goods. Our troops were having to encounter many insurgency tactics, booby traps, tunnels wired with explosives, panji traps, etc.

You know how much I miss you and the kids. Please never quit loving me. I could not do this duty without the love you send in your letters and knowing that I exist in your heart. Hug the kids for me real tight. We are a good family who loves each other and loves the Lord. I can now only picture you with my mind; but, someday, I will hold you again and tell you a million times how much I love you.

Bob

The love that blossomed during my tour in Vietnam was not limited to just us. It was the extravagant love affair of a family. It enlarged our understanding of God's love for us as His adopted children and gave new meaning to our grafted family of five. We loved each other and we were purposed to be together whether born of flesh and blood or adopted. Our family was the result of something greater. It was born of the Spirit, God's vision for us as participants in His great mission. For Jeanette it was that beautiful—even miraculous— moment when motherhood was fully realized in her heart, and through all its challenges and tender moments, motherhood was solidified in her personhood. This personhood would later characterize the essence of her ministry to so many others...

> *The love that blossomed during my tour in Vietnam was not limited to just us.*

October 3, 1966

Bob,

I was so happy when I read your letter today. You talked about wanting to have another child. If you were with me, I would gladly want another baby. After my period of sickness was over, I would be so happy at the thought of being pregnant. When I thought of caring for a little booger like the three we already have, I got so excited. For years, prior to having Dale, I felt like I did not have a right to be called mother by David and Jonne. However, when I became pregnant with Dale, I felt complete and whole. Then, I really felt like a mom to all three of the children. It was as if they became really mine. It was as if now I have a right to be the mother that I always wanted to be. That may seem strange, but it was personal for me to want to be pregnant, as if that was the final mountain to climb to be called that sacred word, "Mother."

With Loving Kisses,

Jeanette

October 18, 1966

My Sweetheart,

I love you so much. I'm so lonesome without you. I do not care how hard I work or how I keep my mind busy, I never cease to think of you: what you're doing; are you safe; will we ever come back together again? I would love so much tonight to be held in your arms and loved until we both fell asleep. It seems like dream stuff to think of our past together. It seems so long ago since I held you close and we made love together. In fact, the 2 ½ months that you've been gone from me seems almost longer than the 18 years that we have been married. We should feel like we are in the middle of our marriage after 18 years, but because I love you so much, it is as if we just got married a couple of years ago. I wish I could settle on the age of 25 and keep us there.

Our three little Indians miss you as much as I do. They still pray for you every day. Dale gets stuck like a broken record asking the Lord over and over again to bring you home safely. Last night at the Krystal he kept praying for you over and over again before he ate his waffle. The people there could not get over him praying so loud and, yet, so tiny, sitting on a big stool, and eating like a big boy. He is a tiny one. It is difficult for me to see him as so small because his mind is so sharp. Really, he is a little rascal. Do you remember how distant he used to be? He did not want to be held, loved, or kissed. Well, he isn't like that anymore. Maybe it's because he's been sleeping with me since you have been gone, and he's gotten used to someone being near him. Now, he likes for me to hold him and rock him to sleep.

Please, take care of yourself.

Jeanette

November 15, 1966

Dearest Jeanette, my Sweetheart (and my three tigers)

Your last letter was a "treasure." I must have read it a dozen times after all lights out. In the silence of the night, I pictured in my mind my beautiful bride caring for those precious ones. It is those images that keep me going, day in and day out, through unbelievable injuries and loss of lives. Otherwise, I think I would lose my mind.

This has been a difficult time. In one parachute jump, I landed right in the middle of a hostile village. Then, the heat has been almost unbearable at times. Everyday seems a repeat of the previous day: long, difficult operations in terrain I never thought even existed, much less us having to cut our way through day in and day out. Then, there is the anxiety of waiting, watching, and anticipating the next crisis. There is good news, though. Men, seasoned Sky Soldiers (nickname for 173rd troops), have been coming in large numbers to our field worship services, giving their hearts to the Lord. And, would you believe it? Baptism services wherever we could find a river that would allow us to baptize these new converts. Your love for me, and your love and care for the kids, strengthen me for this call and mission of the Lord. I feel so unworthy of having received from you so much love and commitment. Please keep that love coming; it is a reminder of why the Lord put us together. Hug and kiss the kids. I miss them and you more deeply each day of this separation.

Bob

In going back, we better understood how we arrived in the place we were. Not in terms of an undisclosed disease but in our relationship. We found our way to this moment because we understood very early that God orchestrated our love and commitments to one another. There was no other fit for our personalities, ministries, and every other part of us that must connect correctly in order to remain faithful for over sixty years. These are the unique attributes which bound us together with cords that could not be broken—unified in mind, body, and spirit. These stories brought to life again, through a collection of dusty letters, the anchors which held us steady when life shifted underneath us like sand in a sand storm. These records of our love and God's faithfulness were our—my—defense when disillusioned by the shiftiness of Alzheimer's. In this next letter, Jeanette rightly calls out these truths—truths which navigated me through the impending life circumstances that would lead to my own moments of disillusionment as we journeyed together to and then through the land and language of Alzheimer's.

October 9, 1966

Bob,

We just came from church. Another one was baptized in the Holy Spirit. That makes three this week. (A friend shared with me this week her struggles as a Christian seeking God and trying to attend church faithfully with a spouse who is adamantly against it.)[26] I was sad because she has to live that way. She is such a fine person.

God gave me a different person, a fine wonderful person. I can lovingly call him my husband. He knew I needed someone like you to take care of me, because I don't get along well with people. If you didn't put up with me, I'd be left out in the cold. I needed you, so God made it possible for us to meet and get married soon afterwards. I had special prayer for you at church tonight. I feel that God has a special work for you and is going to watch over you. That is my constant prayer. So just trust God, and do what you can to proclaim His Word. I'm sending you a new Bible as a special gift just

---

26 The names and details of this story have been removed to respect the privacy of our good friend.

for you being so sweet to me. Be sweet and please take care of yourself. We love you so much until it hurts.

Jeanette

Christmas Day, 1966

Dearest Jeanette:

I must get this to you on this very special Christmas Day. I can only imagine the kids, opening their gifts, and the looks upon their faces when they got that very special thing they had asked and prayed for. You were always so good at getting each of them that very special toy or item. Where did you get such sensitivity? I love you for this and a million other reasons. Earlier today, with the help of two anointed NCO's, I baptized some 35 new converts, won to the Lord over the last few weeks. You cannot imagine the joy we had as each of these new converts gave a brief testimony of their new relationship with the Lord. These two lay preachers danced both in and out of the water. I had to ask them to cool it until we could get all baptized. Our security unit, commanded by one of our young officers, was going crazy trying to hasten up the event, knowing that at any moment a crisis could occur. But, we got through it without any incidents; praise to the Lord. May we never again be separated at Christmas. I love you and hope to spend the rest of my life proving it. Hug the

*kids, and tell them Dad wanted to be there. I can only hope
someday they will forgive me for missing such a special day.*

Bob

In other ways, these letters prepared us for the inevitable separation that comes to every married couple, death. Reading these letters near the end of our lives, together, gave them new meaning. When Jeanette read about the pain of separation, my heart—though full of gratitude for her extravagant love for me—was pierced by the knowledge that someday one of us would experience the anguish of separation, again. Even now these realities—layer by grievous layer —are still unfolding before me. I'm still awakening to her absence in every new routine and every new assignment I take on without her support and wisdom. In a very real way, even as we sat together in our room reading and rehearsing, these last two letters, records of our love, too well documented the difficulties of being separated from one another forcing us—consciously and subconsciously—to consider life without the other.

May 29, 1967

Bob,

*As I awoke this morning, it was so peaceful and quiet. It was
already warm. I wondered if you wished you could wake up
in a quiet and peaceful surrounding. I sometimes ache for
you because I love you so much. When I do not hear from*

you my heart breaks. If you're coming home to us around July 23rd, that means I have to wait painfully for a couple more months. I know that the Lord will help me in my waiting, but I get so excited when I think about that day when your plane arrives, and you come back home to us. I will never forget you boarding the plane for Vietnam. My heart shattered, but I couldn't let you see it. I forced a smile and hid my tears behind my sun glasses. I did not want to break knowing that you had that long, painful flight from here to Vietnam. You had so much on you; leaving us and then going back to Combat. I had to be brave, yet my tears kept coming. I could not stop them. Nobody knows what a wife feels when she knows that she is sending her husband back to a place of the unknown. I feel guilty that I didn't spend every waking moment with you before you left. Who knows, when you come home, I have been thinking about us having another child. At times, I think I am still that girl of 20 when we married. Forgive me for these dreams; they come because I miss you so much.

Please, be careful and remember we love you so very much!

Jeanette

June 12, 1967

Bob,

I'm so lonely today, and no letter came from you. I'm so used to hearing from you every day. I'm worried about your safety. When I don't hear from you, I get pain in my chest, thinking something may have happened. My sweetheart, you're supposed to be back with us in 45 days. It has been 365 days since you left us. I've missed you every one of these days. It's been so lonely without you. There are times when I'm so lonely I think that life is not worth living without you. Only when you're back at home with us will our days seem to really be complete. Our little ones will be so happy when you come home and even more so for their mother; I'm so anxious for my man to come home to me. You are what keeps us going because we care so much for you.

Please, be careful and remember we love you so very much!

Jeanette

June 24, 1967

Dearest Jeanette:

I miss you so much, but, today, like I've never experienced before. I must share with you my pain. I trust you will keep this letter confidential. In fact, if reviewed, it could be "censored." You have most likely read of the event named, "the Battle of the Slopes," just a few miles from our base camp at Dak To / Kontum. One of our companies—a company I had a worship service with just a few days ago, men I know so well, many of them having gotten saved in that recent worship service—experienced one of the most tragic situations I have seen during my time in Vietnam. In a span of just a day or so, this one company engaged with a much larger regiment of regular North Vietnamese soldiers, and in the process we lost 72 soldiers in a company of only 140. I am writing this letter looking out at the large tent where their remains lie in body bags, row after row, thinking, "These young men, sons, have parents back home who have yet to be notified of this tragic loss." You have probably already read this in the newspapers. Ordinarily, I would not write to you about this type of event, but my heart just could not stand the hurt without sharing it with someone I so love and so trust, someone whose prayers mean everything to me. Please forgive me for unloading this on you, especially since I only have another month until I deploy back home. Today, more than ever, I long for your love, understanding, and your confidence in the Lord Jesus. I need to alert you that I will be coming home with a broken heart even with guilt for leaving these young soldiers, who are such a part of our chaplaincy outreach. Many of those that died were carrying a card that we give to new converts, called The Sky Soldier's Christian Fellowship Pledge. This is their formal pledge, after conversion, to walk faithfully with the Lord and to be a strong witness of His Love and Grace with fellow soldiers. I love you and the kids

109

*more than I could ever express. Pray for me and especially our
unit whose grief can be felt throughout our entire base camp.*

Bob

I am so thankful the Lord let Jeanette sense the time to be short;
otherwise, we would have never taken the time to revisit such precious
memories, memories that would be a necessary resource in facing our
future with Alzheimer's disease. The reaffirming fact is that before the
Lord takes us on our penultimate journey, in this case our Alzheimer's
journey, He equips and prepares us. In the typical fashion of Yahweh,
He rehearses the stories of old while intertwining them with our
present as a way to more fully understand His purposes or at least trust
in His presence no matter what comes our way. So, as we examined
our present by retracing our past, we found the Spirit compelling us
forward and upward to newly revealed but ever so difficult destinies.

Who would have thought that our sacred stories, packed away in a
box in our basement, could have had such a profound impact on our
relationship and our journey? To simply deem them a timely find is to
not understand their worth at all. To us they were expressions of God's
selection and unfailing love for His people, our enduring and growing
love for each other, and how those stories gave us the reassurance that
He has a plan for us that goes beyond our life on this good earth. Later
they became markers, road signs, which kept us on a singular path and
purpose, together. Reminders that we were gifted an inseparable love.

Chapter 6

Sacramental Cleansing As Submission, Not Resignation:

Early Phase[27]

The next great wave of change came in 2008. At the time, Jeanette was serving as the Finance and Hospitality Coordinator of the Church of God Chaplains Commission where I had been the Executive Director for 32 years. Together we

---

27 The traditional way to categorize the progression of Alzheimer's disease is to do so through three primary stages: early, middle, and late phase. While these act as a guide, the actual experience is not so easily categorized. One of the problems is that most people live with the disease for years before they are diagnosed. Thus, once diagnosis is made, the recipient may be further along in the progress than expected. For my purposes, these phases act more as indicators of major changes both physically and spiritually in our journey. They are not intended to be perfect identifiers of the disease's progression.

helped to found the Commission. Consequently, the hundreds of chaplains who came up under our leadership had become our many sons and daughters in the faith. This spiritual family was beautifully diverse—male, female, black, white, Hispanic, Asian, etc. —and bound by a common passion for ministry and God. Our commitments and love for one another were mutual: we claimed those chaplains as uniquely ours and they claimed us as the same. Jeanette, their spiritual mother, relished in her honored position. She knew them all, their stories, their needs, their families, their faces. And it was her struggle to recall *their* faces which flagged us that another wave of crisis was mounting.

As we were preparing for the 2008 General Assembly (the bi-annual international ministers' meeting for the Church of God denomination), Jeanette began to have problems managing all of her responsibilities as conference coordinator for the chaplains' events. Though she had been a terrific manager of these activities over the years, this early wave of Alzheimer's made the process more and more difficult for her. She became conflicted and disorganized. The stress of her internal struggle to maintain a professional level of organization led her to become greatly distressed and anxious. I could sense it in her voice. Suddenly what she had done for years so naturally was now taxing and arduous. Yet it was not her nature to relent; she refused to give up those responsibilities which had given her a deep sense of pride. She loved her work and those she was privileged to serve through that work. It was as much a part of her as her own personality or finger print. To give it up was to ask her to give up a portion of who she was. So I covered her. Please don't mistake my words as covering *for* her; rather, we *covered her* keeping her most vulnerable self hidden from the harshness of her new and growing reality.

I think it was at this point that I began to work at being a genuine presence in Jeanette's journey with this disease. I practically camped out in her office, determined that in this not-yet-named journey we would protect her *almost* perfect offerings of ministry and work. We worked very closely together during this time which was not our norm. She did not understand initially my presence, but eventually accepted my companionship as a natural part of her work environment. As I reflect on that time, I now know this was the beginning of my new call: partnering with Jeanette for this journey. The entire office and staff at the Chaplains Commission were enlisted to assist me in this covert operation. Together we were watchful of Jeanette as her health continued to decline causing her work to suffer. She missed things she never would have missed before; sometimes she even mismanaged a major task. Jeanette had carried us in our chaplaincy and seminary activities for over 30 years, often as a volunteer or simply an underpaid worker; now my entire staff assisted me in covering her. We did so not for fanfare or accolades but because we loved and valued those we journeyed with. She wasn't just *my* family; she was their family, too. Therefore we were determined that, regardless of what we had to do, she would maintain a sense that she was successfully completing the tasks she so treasured.

Although a struggle to get there ready and prepared, the 2008 General Assembly came with great excitement. As was customary for our chaplains after checking into their hotels, they made their way to first see their spiritual mother, Jeanette. They came in multitudes with hugs and stories of their families and ministries. Jeanette's ability to handle such occasions with grace and etiquette was never more evident for those who could see *behind the veil*. She miraculously found ways to navigate around the gaps in her memory which kept her from truly knowing those persons in front of her. She called them by name when possible and would lead them toward a more familiar shared story to not give away her failing connections. Of course, when she did struggle to remember, she was given assistance from either one of my staff members or me who waited faithfully by her side. It was her call and vocation to mother those chaplains, and we were intent on creating a space where she could continue in that vocation, well.

In other areas, our sacred covering had to be offered in other ways. As her mind continued to deteriorate, it no longer became safe for her to drive. Other tasks soon followed. Things as simple as balancing her checkbook, losing personal items, completing work on time, or just the repetition of the same stories became indicators that she could no longer manage her duties effectively. Before long, maybe too long, she finally admitted that it was time for her to retire. Her younger sister, Geri, replaced her. Almost miraculously, Jeanette walked her sister through every detail of the office she was leaving, and left her extensive notes concerning this very complicated work. Yet she could no longer do the work herself.

Before we knew it, the 2010 General Assembly was upon us. This one would mark the end of a long and wonderful journey in the development of our chaplaincy ministries around the world.

After thirty-two years, I retired as Director. Hundreds of our chaplains, their families, and our extended church family made this an unforgettable retirement celebration. The participants blessed us with gifts, letters of appreciation, and with their testimonies. They wrote and spoke of Jeanette's great influence, as a spiritual mother, on their lives through her dedicated love and care for them. The last night of our celebration, Jeanette and I met with our chaplains for the last time as the "head" of our chaplaincy family. That night my family took center stage. My kids spoke and shared their experiences living in the Crick home with such a large, extended family. We shared excerpts from reel-to reel recordings of our family correspondences and prayers. We laughed, we cried, we held tight—ever so tight to a life we loved and knew—knowing we had to let go. I too spoke, but for me the Key Speaker was Jeanette. We weren't even sure that she would be able to speak or would still want to speak. Then, with much anticipation, Jeanette took the stage with me just a small distance from her. As much as I wanted her to take her "final bow," I also wanted to keep her safe with me at my side. On that stage she was fully vulnerable and exposed. There would be no one to cover her missteps. My heart raced. I poised myself to be at her immediate disposal.

Looking out over that audience into the multitude of faces, I was reminded of our struggle to conceive and how much Jeanette longed to be a mother. Watching her give her farewell speech, I was overcome by God's ability to satisfy that need both literally and spiritually. She was indeed a mother of many. Though many times in her early years as a mom she struggled to own that identity, on that day, in that moment, through *their words* and *their responses*, it was apparent that she had mastered this great honor. I was so privileged to live it out alongside her and to stand with her as she said her good-byes. Her speech was short but moving. She spoke with meaning and with tears of sincere appreciation for her chaplaincy family. Yet even in her grace, it was apparent that she was losing touch with her memories of these blessed sons and daughters. Shortly after her address, she retreated to her hotel room with notable signs of confusion about "the event" and the meaning of "that dinner."

We weren't the only ones who noticed changes. My children saw it, too, but all of us saw it in different ways...

> *I had definitely noticed some changes in Mom. I had asked her to write a story about her life because I knew she wouldn't be here forever. I wanted to capture her life before it was too late. I remember asking her once if she was writing it, and she told me she had started and reflected back on a story of receiving a red rocker from her Papa (grandfather) as a child. It couldn't have been more than 2 weeks later when she told me that story again. I didn't say anything to her at the time, because I figured she had just forgotten that she told me, but then I started noticing this type of thing happening more and more. She probably told me the rocker story 15 times over the next year or so. Sometimes I listened as if it was the first time and sometimes I tried to help her remember that she had already told me the story. In the end, I dismissed it. She was getting older, and she had a right to forget things from*

time to time. To me, she still seemed mentally sharp. She was still going in to work every day, would talk to me about my children and give me advice. Even at the General Assembly, I didn't see any major changes. Yes, she was tired most of the time and interacted less than usual; but, again, I wrote that off as an issue of age.

—Dale Crick, youngest son

Signs of mom's disease began to surface in various places, such as, retelling stories over and over, misplacing her keys and purse, or having the inability to do the most mundane tasks. Mom had always been very sharp, mentally, but there was something very different. At times we would just attribute this to her aging and maybe slight dementia.

In August 2010, the entire family assembled in Orlando to attend Dad's retirement ceremony at the 2010 General Assembly. It was an opportunity for us to celebrate the many years of service Mom and Dad had given to the church, to chaplaincy families, students and other ministries around the world. It seemed everyone was there. Even the extended family members came to celebrate this momentous event. But internally, I knew Mom was not herself. That whole week, she was very reclusive and did not adapt well to being around a lot of people. She constantly felt bad and resisted leaving her suite. Despite so many people wanting to see her, we felt we needed to limit her visitors so as not to overwhelm her.

Mom did make it to the retirement celebration, though the large crowd of faces unnerved her a bit. Each of us kids worked hard to put together a media presentation on the life and ministry of the Crick family. Mom was there, partially. But, it was very evident it was a major undertaking to have her be there. While many rejoiced as she addressed that vast audience, I knew deep down this was not the same woman who had given so much to this ministry. Something was very different and I only wanted to protect her like she had protected me for so many years.

—Jonne Crick, daughter

I was given the honor of participating in the retirement ceremony for Dad at the General Assembly. I brought with me a truck load of photo albums, slides, journals, a camera, and some computer equipment. Set up in the office space of Mom and Dad's suite, I sifted through years of history— audio recordings, photos and slides, newspaper clippings and Church of God articles—to put together a comprehensive presentation of their ministry. Mom sat with me, working for long hours, as she had done so many times in my life (working endless nights together balancing financial statements for the seminary; assisting me with many term papers;

and taking care of me when I had pneumonia). However, this time was different. As I asked her about the photos and slides, I realized more and more that she could not recall the people in the photos or where the photos had been taken. I also noticed she would tell me the same stories over and over. Then, the night of Dad's retirement ceremony my eyes were opened. When Mom was presented with a gift for her years of faithful service, she was dumbfounded. For just a moment, a lingering awkward moment, she looked at me like she had no idea where she was, why she was there, or why she was getting a gift. I left there heartbroken. I couldn't imagine my Mom in such a weakened state. She had always been so strong for all of us; it was unimaginable to see her now so fragile.

——David Crick, oldest son

The Transforming Nature of the Disease: Not by Might, Nor by Power, but by [His] Spirit

Retirement is a major shift in anyone's life. I'm not sure that I was fully ready or even fully wanted to retire. I loved my position and the many Kingdom opportunities that the job provided. In many ways our individual and shared identity was in chaplaincy ministry. While Jeanette was slipping away from that identity I was still grasping for it fully aware of, yet denying, its fleeting presence.

Overcome by the transitions in my life, denial—maybe even avoidance—became my primary way to cope with these changes. I didn't want to accept or see the obvious playing itself out in front of me —I was no longer the Director of the Chaplains Commission and my wife was embarking on the battle of her life. Activity willingly fed my avoidance, as it often does. Instead of closing the door to that old life I kept it propped open through part-time teaching at the seminary and working with my dearest and closest friend, Tom, on some international projects. But when the Lord intends a door to be closed He will make it shockingly clear. A horrific event that couldn't be avoided happened. Tom suddenly died due to a massive heart attack. He and his wife, Elaine, were avid supporters of our chaplaincy ministry and partnered with us on several other projects. Tom's death knocked me into the reality of my present situation and led me to refocus and accept Jeanette's journey as my journey, too.

> *I could again hear the Lord saying, "Bob, this is the life I have for you. You must learn not only to tolerate it, but embrace it."*

The Lord had already spoken to me in the previous year that her change would also bring about a major change in me. With the jarring realities of Tom's death, I could again hear the Lord saying, "Bob, this is the life I have for you. You must learn not only to tolerate it, but embrace it."

I experienced this Word only in part, as is often true with Divine Revelation. Paul describes this phenomenon in 1 Corinthians 13: 12, albeit he was describing revelation in terms of eschatology, "*For now we see in a mirror dimly, but then face to face. Now I know in part; then I shall know fully, even as I have been fully known.*" Please give me the leeway to make my application, though limited in its scope. Like a dimly lit mirror, my sight or understanding of what was unfolding in my heart was limited. In other words, I could clearly see that something was there, but could not see that something clearly. Yet…eventually…I would meet that something face-to-face. No longer an image in the mirror or a reflection of things to come. One day that image would become a tangible part of my life. I could no longer deny what was before me.

You see, that revelation gave to me "knowledge in part," a knowledge that would unfold and become more focused in time. Even now, looking back with a better vantage point—a more clarifying line of vision—I realize I do not, yet, fully know. But I will someday, as certain as I know that I am fully known by Him. Where am I at in that process a year after her death? I know in full that the Lord used her disease to extend to me His "Sacrament of Cleansing." The life He had prepared for me, through her journey, was a cleansed life free from that extra baggage I had accumulated over my 50 years of ministry in two very difficult and demanding agencies: the military and general church ministries. I was being retooled and refocused for what has proven to be the most transformational season of my life's call and vocation. My new call, my new assignment, at that time was to join Jeanette on her journey into this strange and new land of Alzheimer's Disease. Eventually that journey would extend outward to include our children, not just cleansing me, but mercifully transforming me and my family in the process.

In the early part of this journey, the Lord showed me through a dream that this process would indeed be my epiphany. That defining phase of my life would initiate a change which would reach the very core of my mind and soul, forever changing me! Time and again my mind would wander back to Jeremiah 29:11 as a comforting reminder that God's plans are good plans. The process is a struggle, but he never abandons us to the process. He is perpetually immersed in it with us and for us. Because His eyes are ever on a hope-filled future. He never leaves. He never forsakes. Always compels us forward in our pressing toward that *already, not yet* prize found in the person and promises of Jesus Christ.

> *The process is a struggle, but he never abandons us to the process.*

Did these Words of Truth minimize my struggle? Not a chance. Did I continue to struggle with this major shift in principle and practice of my identity, both personally and vocationally? Of course. I initially tried to hold on to segments of the old. But my spirit-man kept telling me to let go of all of those time and energy consuming passions of my previous vocation—those "loves" of my life. The Lord had taken me all over this world to minister on His behalf, and now He was planting us at home for a very important new call and ministry. Although it didn't seem as important at the time. In truth, it felt like a time out. There was no pomp and circumstance, no awe and wonder. Just stuck in a terminal unable to take flight. I thought He had clipped my wings, when in reality he was unloading all the unnecessary weight—a hollowing out of that which kept me grounded.[28] The Lord was cleansing me in order that He might recreate me in His image, not the one fashioned after the world of "office" and "man's systems," heavy and burdened. Rather, the one emptied of this world and filled with the hallowed breath of God. Like birds set to flight, we were meant to be *hollowed out* so that we might mount up with wings as eagles at His appointed time. He was using this painful process to do just that. In the end, the extent to which I accepted this new call would determine how deep the cleansing—the *hollowing*—would affect me personally and to what extent the *hallowing* would be transformational.

Unplugging from my known world wasn't just a philosophical idea or spiritual twist on a good story. It was a reality. It was my experience lived out through retirement, loss of friends and vocation, and the failing health of Jeanette. On top of all of this, we moved 130 miles away from our Tennessee residence of 34 years—the hub of all those offices and systems—to Georgia (outside of my known life) to be near our children and grandchildren. I felt alone and distanced from a life I loved and a community from which I drew support. In an attempt to maintain some measure of that old life I found ways to stay connected. I continued to teach part-time at our seminary a couple days per week until eventually, Jeanette's

---

28 One of the four forces which allow birds to take flight is their weight—or lack of weight. Everything from their wings to their beaks create opportunity for flight. Among those are hollowed bones which allow them to be light enough to fly. Spiritually speaking, our waiting on the Lord in these seasons of transition is really a transformation. It is the hollowing out of all the baggage and systems which weigh us down. Thus, mysteriously, in the waiting our strength is renewed, and we are transformed from ground dwellers to eagles that soar.

disease progressed into its advanced stages. Thankfully, the Lord was merciful and patient with me in this transformation. His plans were greater than my avoidance and resistance. His plans anticipated the mountains which I created, yet needed to level. More than anything else, His plans anticipated the measure of compassion and encouragement I would need to allow this transformation to occur.

In the midst of all this external change, Jeanette's situation was quickly progressing. The changes were becoming more obvious. Changes that marked a turning point from simply those initial symptoms to more progressed symptoms. While many of the changes were expected, some were unexpected and humorous. Jeanette suddenly became very protective of our dog Skipper. Unlike the "earlier Jeanette" who never wanted a dog in the house she now became inseparable with Skipper. He was given an elevated status in our house, the object of her affections. She constantly held on to him, feeding him his regular meals with lots of in between snacks. If I tried to discipline Skipper in any manner, she would immediately come to his defense. He became one of her most important stabilizing anchors as Alzheimer's destroyed more and more of her memories, language abilities, and her emotions. She once even got lost with Skipper—at least, lost from us. In her mind she most certainly was not lost. She and Skipper just decided to go for an afternoon walk...without telling anyone...on their own. After a frantic search which included the local police department, family and neighbors, she was found with Skipper following along beside her, walking around casually, unaware of all the commotion at her expense. While it almost scared me into an early grave, I can now look back with a smile. Her identity never changed; she was independent and headstrong. She always knew what she wanted and did it. That day was no different, except that she was radically unaware of her own impairments in judgment… .

Not all of her changes were as humorous and fulfilling as her newly blossoming relationship with Skipper. The advancement of the initial phase brought loss for Jeanette, also. Some of Jeanette's beloved interests became too difficult for her to continue. She loved to trace down her family's history. She had files of genealogical materials dating back hundreds of years. In the earlier days we would visit old graveyards, libraries, courthouses and all the other places which store these old historical documents. She never surrendered to any challenges. However, like so many interests, this well ingrained habit also lost its place in her fading memories. Finally, she agreed to pass on her many sacred findings to other family members.

She always knew what she wanted and did it. That day was no different; except that she was radically unaware of her own impairments in judgment.

Jeanette was, also, an avid reader—an appreciation she developed as a child. She loved to read classic novels, historical books and Christian novels. As the disease continued to disable more and more of her cognitive faculties, reading became more difficult than she could bear. She would get stuck on a page, reading words and sentences over and over. Frustrated, she would just give up and try later. Eventually later wasn't worth the struggle, and she gave up reading altogether. Nonetheless, this desire never left her. Knowing she could no longer read these beloved books, she would simply cling to them. Often I would find her holding a book tightly to her chest, like she was clinging to a fading memory to the very end. The overflow of this issue was most pronounced in her daily devotions; Jeanette loved to read the Word of God more than any other book. Faithfully, for more than twenty-five years, she read through the entire Bible each year wearing out several Bibles in the process. Inside the columns of her Bibles she would record family prayer needs, birthdays, and insights on how a particular scripture applied to her relationship with the Lord. As her condition worsened, the severity of her symptoms no longer allowed her to complete this daily discipline. Wanting to help her in any way I could find (to both overcome her feelings of helplessness and defeat mine as her helpmate), I felt it was my duty to keep alive this discipline for both of our sakes. Daily I read to her following her strict reading plan, almost right up to her death. When she would fall asleep, I kept on reading. I was determined in this and so many other areas of her life to be her behind the scenes substitute. On my own, I can't imagine how difficult it was for her to hand over such beloved acts. Her surrendering of interests was not simply her giving up some novel pursuit; she was giving up pieces of herself. They were acts and pursuits that she had cultivated and loved. They were the details that made up the unique mosaic of her personhood. All of it collectively made her my Katherine Jeanette Crick.

While our world was drastically changing, some things remained the same. We did what we had done for many years. We went for short walks (with Skipper in tow). We talked about life, our kids and grandkids. And, we talked about us—our love and our life together. Knowing there would come a day, very soon, when she might be uncomfortable with me hugging her, I hugged her as often as I could. We also prayed together, regularly. This is where I found the Spirit's encouragement and strength for the more difficult days. Her prayers were often wrought with disconnected phrases; but, for me, prayer was the one stabilizing force that never left Jeanette. Even as she advanced into the latter stages of her disease, she loved to pray. She prayed long series of prayers, sometimes praying herself to sleep.

In looking back, I better understand now that Jeanette's "surrenderings" were submissions; they were never resignations. She never resigned herself to the disease, giving up like one without hope. Rather, she led us in submitting ourselves to God's greater purposes for her last great chapter on this earth. In truth, it was she who first showed me how to submit to the changes. Watching her hand over her independence, her personal interests and hobbies, even the disciplines of her faith to me, to others, and most importantly to the Lord was one of the most humbling encounters of my life and my ministry formation. In spite of her own fears and struggles with the disease, it was she who could more clearly see through the mountains that I wanted leveled. It was then

> *I better understand now that Jeanette's "surrenderings" were submissions; they were never resignations.*

I better understood our roles. She had to be our guide and our teacher. And we had to follow her.

The irony of our journey was that Jeanette was the least likely candidate to lead us. It was almost illogical to conceive of such a strategy. Yet in spite of her many growing deficiencies, she was the one who could see. So I trusted in her spiritual sight as we (our family) followed closely by faith. In the process, we discovered that the more willing we were to follow her lead and submit to these new realities, the greater our chances were to remain on the journey with her a little longer and to be changed by that journey with her. It was as if we were players in the old Christian classic, *Hinds' Feet in High Places*.

Like the central figure, we weren't sure if we could make the climb. But we were certain that God was with us, leading and directing, even strengthening us for the climb as we learned to enlarge our Trust in him. We were experts at trusting the Lord with our minds, but trusting him with our hearts—even with a long Pentecostal history—is a steep and cumbersome climb. The Word which ran so richly through the very chemistry of our lives became our guide, particularly passages like Proverbs chapter 3:5-6 (NKJV), "Trust in the Lord with all your heart, and lean not on your own understanding; in all your ways acknowledge Him, and He shall direct your paths." As our trust in Him enlarged, so did our acknowledgements of His presence and providence. We in a sense gave God the nod; by faith, we saw Him at work and trusted His work to be Good and necessary. More than that, acknowledging Him was vouching for Him, willfully putting our own names on the line for His name's sake. In the acknowledging of His ways we found ourselves better able to submit to His direction, for we knew we were indeed, at His mercy. When that happens (for any of us!), He promises to make our paths straight (NIV). I'm not suggesting He is going to give us an easy path without all the twists and turns that come with the trek. This is not true. Rather, a straight path is an indication of God's sovereignty as the One who will surely bring us to an appointed goal, His goal. The certainty that God had a specific, appointed goal gave us the strength to journey even in the most difficult places with her longer. A goal He would more fully disclose after her death.

The Climb: From Foothills to Mountain Ranges

Obviously, Jeanette had little choice in what she became as the disease took its toll. But we always had the choice to "tap out." The steeper the climb the more difficult it was to keep our commitments. Our commitments were commitments of love, yet not always out of understanding. This is the way it is with most people I suppose. We are "all in" from the beginning.; then the increasing struggles enter the picture. Suddenly the commitments strain our lives tempting, sometimes forcing, us to reconsider what those commitments look like. Self says there is no way to fulfill them; we are foolish and naïve to think we can. Self reminds us of days when things were easier and offers solutions that would let us "off the hook." To protect our fragile egos we carefully and craftily rename this self as self-preservation rather than calling it what it is: selfishness.

You see, speaking in general, we enter in not fully understanding how these new commitments fit into an already existing lifestyle. Since most of us aren't good at restructuring our lives to fit yet another task into the mix, we are fully unprepared for the daunting job of caring for a person who has a debilitating disease such as Alzheimer's disease. Much must be given up in order to accommodate these commitments, including outside relationships. For many of us, we just aren't willing to do it until we have to. As much as we don't want to admit it, we are selfish about our personal agendas and comforts. Having the freedom to pursue or fulfill personal goals is no longer an option; caregivers are left feeling very alone and isolated in their experience.

Inwardly, especially in the early stages, I would cry out, is there anyone out there who knows what I am going through? I felt alone, afraid, and completely helpless. As I considered this unknown future my thoughts would overwhelm me. Everything around me is changing, Lord! My wife is not my wife; she is more like my child. Georgia is not my home. I am detached from my old life, the support of my colleagues, my dialogue partners, and my long term friends. Please, come to my aide. I am lost and afraid. The move, the separation from friends, the changes in Jeanette, and the loss of my ministry and identity became too overwhelming for me. This was the stage where reality relentlessly pursued me. While difficult, it was the most necessary stage because it forced me beyond an awakening and into a jarring awareness that my family and I must prepare ourselves, in whatever way necessary, to complete this journey.

Adapting to this new life was so very difficult, possibly my biggest struggle. Maybe because there was too much change in my life at once. It was as if I once had the opportunity to manage a 10,000-acre farm with lots of good equipment and lots of support personnel, then one day without warning or discussion, I was relocated to a new farm—a one-acre farm—with few support staff and even fewer workers. With this "new call" and vocation, I had to learn a new language in a new land, and I had to learn again how to be a simple and focused farmer. The Lord assured me that, if I would be faithful to this new reality, He would supply me with my daily substance in caring for this one very significant person one step at a time. I learned later, as this new identity sunk in, that God was fashioning in me, again, a basic care identity best illustrated in our marriage vows: for better or for worse, for richer, for poorer, in sickness and in health, to love and to cherish, from this day until death do us part. In other words, my most treasured and worthwhile pastoral identity was wrapped up in my role as her husband.

My new call, my new one acre "farm," didn't have much space for all the baggage I brought with me on the journey, nor did I have time to work out the necessary changes which would allow me to unload much of it in order to join her. I had to be willing to look deeply within my own soul and decide once and for all whether this would be my new and primary call. Little did I know that the Lord had a plan greater than I could have ever conceived. He was using Jeanette's Alzheimer's journey as a means by which to creatively take her from this part of His Kingdom to Paradise, and He was using this event as the means by which to cleanse me, my family, and all those who exposed themselves to this process. I know there will be cynics who will reject the elevation of this terrible event to a place of extraordinary power and profound personal significance. Nevertheless, God is a God of love and Kingdom purpose. He is strategic and intentional about all of our life stories. Nothing is outside of His care or handiwork, not even pain, disease, or struggle. It is up to us to see and perceive—even point to—that greater work.

I had to wrestle with the big questions: What does it mean? And, where will it take us? I had to give myself permission to humbly seek the Lord in prayer: Lord, I know you are the Master of all things that affect our lives. So, Lord, why Jeanette? Why let her experience the gradual loss of her memories, her creativity and passions, and, most of all, her connection to her family? Many people who face a crisis decide that these questions are off limits. Maybe they even decide they are not interested in His answers; they just want Him to take it back, to return them to a former, more glorious moment. Yet, for those of us willing to see and hear, His answer is clear: Let me show you. By faith this is what our family negotiated from the very beginning. We wanted to see the Lord in all of it—the good, the bad, and even the most trying. We knew the only way to see Him in it was to stay in the journey with her, to willingly be changed by it, and selflessly bear witness to the whole process.

To remain on the journey authentically was no easy task. At times it was even cyclical: all in, losing steam/purpose, can't take another step or give up another thing, God intervenes and renews our commitments, repeat. I had grown accustomed to certain values, beliefs, and roles. I thought I knew who I was in relation to God and Jeanette but I soon found out that I only knew in part the plan and ultimate role the Lord would give me. As I struggled through a season of soul searching, the Word opened new and wonderful insights for me. I had been in ministry for more than 55 years with numerous positions and responsibilities. Without realizing it, the tensions and strains of these ministries remained with me. I found it very difficult to distance myself from them. In fact, I had no idea how to begin this painful process of shedding off that old life even though I was already experiencing its realities. Still, the tension of those responsibilities lingered within my soul.

I knew I had to find a way to be cleansed from all that I carried for those many years in order to give full attention, with integrity, to Jeanette. That past life was my Goshen[29]—a temporary promise of provision and prosperity. It was supposed to be a place of drawing near. However, somewhere along the way, we decided it would be a place of settling down. Consequently, drawing near morphed into a must remain; I was unknowingly bound to the land of plenty. Though idyllic in its conception, over the years, the burdens of that life had enslaved our hearts. I was too attached to that old baggage to even think of putting it all aside. So I tried hard to keep some near.

This new call and new challenge was very personal. It demanded my full attention and passion. God kept challenging me to look inward and be honest about my condition; I was too overburdened

---

29 Goshen was the area given to the Israelites by Joseph while in Egypt. It was to be a place of honor and provision, a place of nearness to Joseph (Genesis chapters 41-45). Goshen literally means, "drawing near," a fitting name for a family that was being reconciled.

with all those other lingering attachments and passions to turn my full attention to this one person and her journey. I even considered the possibilities of holding on to the old while adding extra responsibilities on to an already overloaded schedule. This was the role I played in life. I was superman; I could do it all. The Lord saw through and rejected these initial negotiations. He would not allow me to make a partial commitment. I could either join her fully and be transformed by it or simply be an observer at a safe distance, untouched by the power of this sacramental cleansing.

The Lord was encouraging me to rid myself of the pretenses of my worldly positions so I could hear anew His call without any "hidden agendas." My initial answer was similar to that of Nicodemus (John 3: 1-21) who asked, "How can a man be born (renewed) when he is old? Can he enter a second time into his mother's womb and be born?" (ESV). As I posed my questions to the Lord in my heart, it was Jesus's answer that I heard so clearly, "Very truly I tell you, no one can enter the Kingdom of God unless they are born of water and the Spirit. Flesh gives birth to flesh, but the Spirit gives birth to spirit" (NIV).

This passage is most often interpreted only in regards to that initial task of being born again. But to me, it is also a universal principal that faces each of us when the Lord moves us from one phase of spiritual maturity to another for our sake and for the Kingdom's. He was saying, "Don't miss this opportunity. Embrace it fully letting go of all those things that inhibit this rebirth, this renewal. Love Jeanette and me at another level and allow us to love you in a way that will teach you what you will need when you too will be asked to take that final journey with me."

Without a doubt, Tom's untimely death had already set me on a course toward healing, but the thing that finally moved me to a deeper and more transformational decision was watching Jeanette be ravaged by this disease, I knew in my heart that if I did not genuinely join her quickly on this journey I would miss the last chapter of our long life and ministry together. In my brokenness, suddenly for the first time in years, I could put all these so called important things—places, events and persons that I had compulsively clung to—in their rightful place. That does not mean they were forgotten forever. No. Goshen was a necessary and God-purposed stop in our greater journey. But those attachments to Goshen (the "leeks and onions" I longed for) no longer held their compulsive power to entice and to enslave. More importantly, I was on a path to follow the Lord as he rearranged my priorities, reminding me the greatest of these priorities was love, my vowed love to Jeanette.

I was on a path to follow the Lord as he rearranged my priorities, reminding me the greatest of these priorities was love, my vowed love to Jeanette.

As things fell into their rightful place, my well-planned maneuvers to keep doing all the things I so cherished in my fifty plus years of ministry began to crumble one by one right before my very eyes. I knew that the Lord was directing this transformational cleansing. He was letting me see the reality of that past life. It was good, but

135

it was never intended to be permanent. I came to realize that the systems of this world are only a means toward a purposed end. Like the Children of Israel in Egyptian bondage, I could hear the Lord instructing, "Don't look back. That old life in Goshen is in the past. Look to the new life that I, the Lord God, will raise up for you and the next generation."

In that place of revelation the Lord spoke ever so clearly to me through Romans 12: 9-13 (NIV), "Love must be sincere. Hate what is evil; cling to what is good. Honor one another above yourselves. Never be lacking in zeal, but keep your spiritual fervor, serving the Lord. Be joyful in hope, patient in affliction, and faithful in prayer. Share with God's people who are in need. Practice hospitality." By faith I knew what I had to do. So I made a faith commitment to a new call and submitted to His tearing away of those burdensome roles and the baggage that came with them. Through His mercy I experienced this as a regeneration, a return to that youthful love of God. Like Gomer,[30] I too chased after my own agenda and desperately needed God to strip me of all those "lovers." In doing so, He led me into the desert. In my aloneness and spiritual/emotional nakedness, He wooed me in the wilderness. There he returned the joy of my youth. In his uprooting of me from those places, I had been

---

30 Gomer is the wife of the prophet Hosea. Hosea was instructed by God to redeem and marry Gomer, a prostitute, who would be unfaithful to him. This was supposed to represent Israel's unfaithfulness to God. In chapter two of Hosea, The Lord strips her of her lovers and all the other external pleasures which kept her attention off of God. Naked and alone, He draws her into the wilderness where she is transformed by his husbandry love. It is the moment when God shifts from master to husband; and it is the moment when she is planted in a more permanent place.

planted, He graciously planted me beside her. And there I came to know Him in a most intimate way. Renewed and seeing with greater clarity, I could more readily empty myself for His refilling and my rebirth. I could receive a new name and mission with a willing heart, as if starting out for the first time in ministry, again. Finally, I was fully joined with her on her journey into the land and language of Alzheimer's.

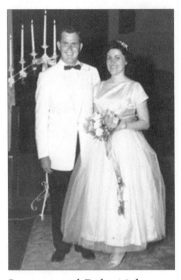

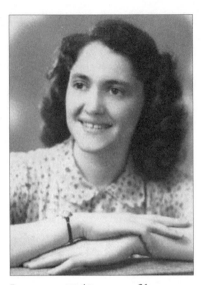

Jeanette and Bob; 10th
Wedding anniversary,
renewal of vows

Jeanette; 1948, year of her
marriage to Bob

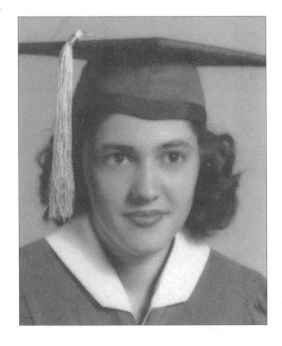

Jeanette; 1946,
graduation from HS

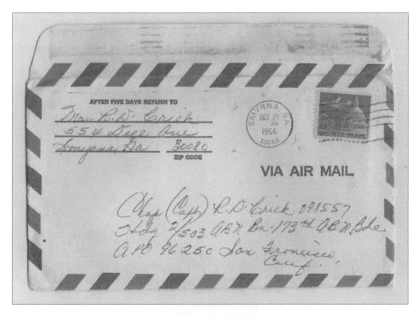

Letter; of the style during Vietnam conflict

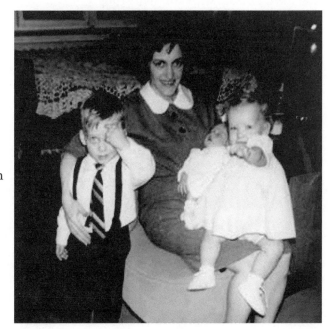

Jeanette with her three children, David, Dale and Jonne; 1964 in Germany

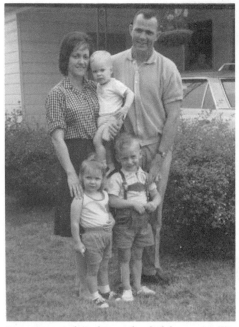

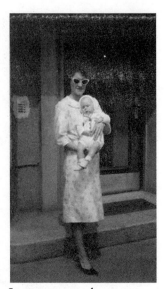

Jeanette; new born,
Dale, 1964, Germany

Jeanette and Bob, with children, 1965
prior to going to Vietnam

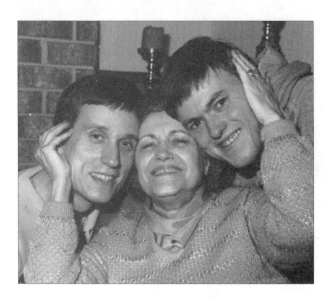

Jeanette
with her two
sons, David
(left) and
Dale (right),
1988

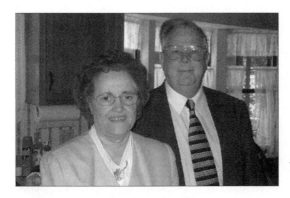

Jeanette and Bob;
Mother's Day, 1998

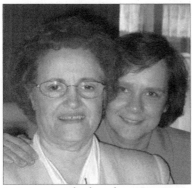

Jeanette with daughter Jonne,
Mother's Day 1998

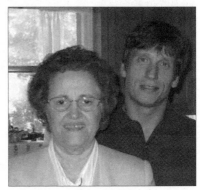

Jeanette with son David,
Mother's day 1998

First grand-
kids of Jeanette
and Bob Crick,
2005

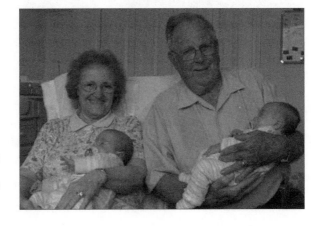

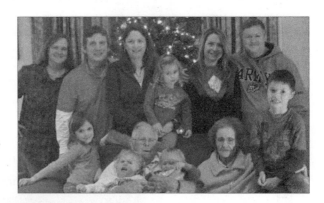

Whole family (11 of us); Jeanette and Bob, children and grandkids, Christmas 2011

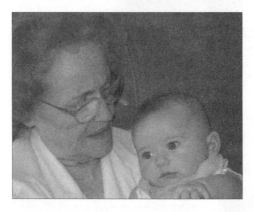

Jeanette with grand-daughter, Samantha, 2009

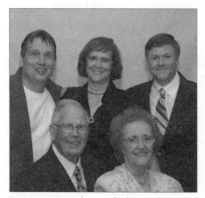

Jeanette, Bob, and their three children, David, Jonne, and Dale; Church Conference 2008

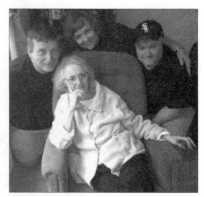

Jeanette, with (left to right) her children, Mother's Day 2014, just months prior to her death

Chapter 7

Middle Phase

No Place like Home:
New Realities Require
New Perceptions

My "awakening" came in March 2011. Prior to that, Mom seemed okay to me. Don't get me wrong; she forgot things and repeated stories, but I would not have considered them major indicators of illness.

Then the undeniable happened. Dad needed to go to Cleveland and asked my wife and me to come with them because he thought there might be a problem with her going back to their Tennessee home. I thought this was kind of silly but agreed because he insisted. We walked into the house and were sitting in the living room when Mom stated, "We better get out of here before the owner of this house returns!" Now Dad had told me about this, but I had never seen it. It was shocking and scary. I had never seen my Mom so confused and afraid. She began to cry and beg to be taken home. In my entire life I had rarely seen my mother cry, and I had never seen her so helpless.

She looked like a lost child begging for help. I really didn't know what to do. I wanted to do anything I could to help her. I begged Dad to take her to a hotel, to Aunt Geri's house or even back to Georgia. Just get her out of that house! This titan of strength that I had relied on my whole life was suddenly broken. The Mom I could confide in; the Mom I could lean on was gone. It was so shocking that it almost felt like a death, I could scarcely recognize this new person.

After that moment, I could never again refute what was happening. My eyes were wide open. It all made sense. My Mom was sick and the person I knew and loved would never come back to me. I would never again share pain or fear with her, I would never again lean on her or seek her advice. Our roles had changed forever…
—Dale Crick

Our Home, Cleveland, TN (March 2011)

Let's leave this house quickly! The owners will find us here, and I don't want to be here when they arrive!"

"Jeanette? What are you talking about? We built this house. This is our home. It's your home."

"Don't you lie to me! I should know my own home. We need to go. They will find us here, and we will be in big trouble!"

"Jeanette, this simply isn't true. We've lived here for 34 years. We raised our kids here. Don't you remember?"

"Please, Bob! We must go. I don't want the owners to find us here. Why can't you see that we must go?"

"Jeanette, you're not thinking straight. You know this place. Dale, tell her."

Dale, confused and scared for his mom, chimed in urging her to listen and trust me, "Mom, he is telling the truth. This is your home, our home."

Insistent that I could convince her, I kept urging her back to our reality, "Come on, I'll show you."

"No! I don't want to go anywhere except out of here, please!"

Again, Dale pleaded, "Mom, just do it. Look around with us, so you can see that this is your house."

Realizing I needed to speak calmly and gently to offset her panic, I took a breath and with my arm gently on her back I assured her, "No one will come. I promise. Just look around with me."

Urging her from room to room, we pointed out anything that might bring her back to her senses. "See, here is the gift we bought you during our vacation in Europe and the pictures we took in Germany and England. These are the scrapbooks you made for our family and puzzles you love to complete. Don't you remember any of it? Look at the pictures on the wall. A stranger wouldn't have *our* pictures on *their* walls. Think about it. This is your house."

Nothing was familiar to her. It was as if she had awakened and found herself in a strange place with almost no recognizable objects. She insisted it wasn't her house. I insisted it was. I was right. She and

I were logical people. If I could just reason with her, I knew I could convince her or at least help her to remember. To remember this was her house, *our house*. The house we built together in 1978, our most permanent home after leaving the military. The house she personally designed and supervised the building of. The house she made sure was ready for our family by Christmas that same year when contractors failed to do their jobs. The house she now perceived to be a strange and fearful building. The house that was no longer home to her.

In her fearful state, she pleaded over and over for our quick departure. Her feelings were real and genuine. Still, I tried my hardest to convince her that my reality of time, place, and people was authentic and hers was distorted. I did so regardless of how she felt. I even tried to explain to her that she was sick and wasn't thinking straight. Naturally, she rejected this rather dogmatic perception.

The more I tried to convince her to stay, the more visibly anxious she became. By this time Dale and Carmen were also visibly shaken by the events. Dale began to plead with me to just take her somewhere else, anywhere else. He hated to see her in such distress. At this point both Dale and Jeanette insisted we leave; I insisted we stay. The whole experience was intense as we all tried to intervene in a situation we truly didn't understand.

Finding ourselves at an impasse, we did what was most natural for us: we prayed. In that prayer, in spite of intense confusion and an incredible fear of things once beloved and familiar, she lifted up a prayer to her rock and anchor, Jesus Christ:

"Oh, Father! We know you are the One and only God. You keep us. You take care of us. So, please be with us tonight. Not just me, but all of us. We depend on you for the strength we so need tonight. Father, we love you with everything in us, and we want you to know that we will do everything we can to keep you in our hearts and to keep your presence with us so that we will always know where we are and who we are. In your love and in your mercy. Amen"

Prayer became our most successful tool in caring for her. Those days which were more difficult or confusing or fearful for her, prayer and singing hymns would bring a necessary relief to her distress. For that moment, a new reality would enter into our presence. As we struggled to find God in the midst of our crisis, the Spirit of the Lord would enter in to our internal chaos dispelling our shared confusion and helplessness. The spirit came to us in so many wonderful ways. Through prophetic utterances and other visitations, He carried us in our desperation toward His transient interventions. These moments were powerful but not daily. On those off days we muddled through the best we could, trusting in His promises of care and sustaining grace.

Perception is Reality

There was certainly no more denial. Jeanette had definitely advanced beyond the initial effects of the disease. It was obvious she needed a more aggressive and long-term treatment plan that would hopefully slow down the damaging effects of the disease. We, as a family, had to finally accept the reality of her new state as she progressed further into this next devastating phase of the disease. As fearful as it was for us, I can only imagine how fearful this process was for Jeanette. To recognize and feel the changes occurring and have no control over them; even more so, to not recognize and understand these uncontrollable changes and experience them so fully as an unknown and uncertain reality. It must have been overwhelming—a repeated and rapidly increasing blow of crushing realities that left her disoriented and confused. As she moved further into this middle phase, she journeyed further and further ahead of us. Faster than we could keep up. Sometimes so far ahead she became unreachable in our present reality.

We knew that once this happened she would never come back to us from that land, so with God's help, we went to her as often as we were able. That became the biggest challenge in the Middle Phase of her Alzheimer's disease journey. The Jeanette of yesterday was fading. Because her body and struggling mind would do anything possible to survive, she began forming new realities which she incorporated into her new "state of mind." Though challenging, we made it our purpose to do whatever necessary to adapt to this new reality so we might accompany her fully on the journey. It wasn't easy, and it wasn't always a nice and forward moving progression. It was more like adjustments—sometimes ever so slight adjustments.

One of the most difficult adjustments was surrendering my own perception of reality for hers. Like so many who initially engage persons with Alzheimer's disease, I fell into that trap of trying to convince Jeanette that her reality was wrong and mine was right. The truth, however, is that persons with Alzheimer's disease lose touch with their homes, their belongings, and their families. In their new state they long and search for that lost state, those things common and familiar and safe. They are separated from their spouse, children, and friends. So they search fearfully, trying to understand and adapt to the "new land" they awaken to with its own internal structures and language—a language *they* speak but most people around them do not. While this is true in part, the greater truth is that we who are able to understand the change refuse to acknowledge its presence and reality.

Jeanette, like most with Alzheimer's disease, adjusted the best she could. She sometimes went along with others' interpretation of her behavior even though her interpretations were often radically different. I'm certain she felt at a disadvantage trying to prove herself to others who had no framework to even discuss these issues with her. As time went on, these episodes of disorientation worsened with less memory to recover. In my crazed perception I was convinced I could persuade her to return to us in spite of the realities of her condition.

I plowed with strength of mind and the power of persuasion without success only to discover it wasn't her false reality that mounted before me; it was mine.

My insistence was really more resistance. More man-made mountains which exchanged her false reality for my false reality. What I wanted more than anything was for her reality to be that leveled mountain prophesied about in Zechariah 4:6. So, I plowed with strength of mind and the power of persuasion without

149

success only to discover it wasn't her false reality that mounted before me; it was mine. She had Alzheimer's, and the life we had known in a land and language familiar to us was gone. I was the one trying to reject our new reality. Ironically, she was more aware of the shift than I was.

Long before any of these things surfaced, the LORD was well at work within me, helping and preparing me. From my clinical experiences to counseling ministry I had gained enough exposure to this disease to know there would be costly adjustments. Even though my intentions were good, I knew I could not succeed on my own. I needed a Rhema Word, that timely revelation of God which gives insight and understanding into a crisis situation. And I got it.... .

When someone is in crisis, their perception is reality. This was the revelation that set me on a path toward freedom and finally released the Spirit of God to level my mountain. It was the insight that allowed me to reclaim a truth I once knew but misplaced, the perception that allowed me to see again the God who had been very kind to us throughout our life, and the truth which granted me access to Jeanette's reality. As much as it went against my logical mind, I had to find a way to accept her reality. And consequently, accept my own. Relinquishing the need to manage the disease, I eventually submitted to the greater reality that this was her journey. A journey she had no control over or choice to decline. If I was going to keep myself attached to her, I must—we must—be willing to follow on her terms and not mine. I would have to be a good follower and a quick learner if I were to keep up. Though difficult beyond words, my kids and I lived as best as we could, in her present reality—whatever that looked like—and prepared ourselves for a more difficult and accepted future.

That acceptance unlocked a more profound experience in my already unconditional love for her. No matter what state she was in, how exhausting or attacking, we loved all of her—old Jeanette and newly evolving Jeanette. We loved her when she would insist she wasn't in her own home, we loved her when she declared we were not her family, and we loved her when she made false accusations about us. We did so by letting go of our need to control the moment and the reality. When she allowed it, we just hugged her lovingly and reassuringly. When she needed it, we drove her around looking for her real home. Occasionally this worked. Most of the time it did not. Never giving up, we tried over and over again.

Plaques & Tangles: Battle for the Brain

As with most Alzheimer's clients, the disease took Jeanette on a rather predictable journey through the various stages of Alzheimer's disease with each stage doing irrevocable brain damage. The middle phase is one of the more difficult phases to witness. This phase is where, despite the loss of brain function, many memories and some skills are still evident. To watch this as her family is like a "wartime scene," an army with weapons described as abnormal protein fragments, Plaques and Tangles, being accumulated in the brain and moving from one section of Jeanette's brain to another.[31] These

---

31 For a more detailed description of this process, see David Shenk's series of web videos at www.aboutalz.org

protein fragments appeared initially in the area of her brain called the hippocampus. This is the area where Jeanette's memories were first born. Therefore, trying to recall something that happened to her after these damaging "movements" became more and more difficult and finally impossible. From this initial afflicted area the plaques and tangles continued to move over a period of time to other areas of the brain.

With noticeable results, after Jeanette's loss of short-term memories, the plaques and tangles moved into the area of her brain where language was processed. Jeanette was particularly astute in both written and spoken language, always noticeably correct and willing to correct others, unlike me, who often butchered the "King's language." Suddenly this bright articulate lady had difficulty forming the right words to express what she was feeling. Being a witness to this change, watching her lose in her struggle for articulation, was painful and heart-sickening to say the least.

This was especially true with someone as independent as Jeanette; even the slight loss of her well-learned abilities became frustrating with outbursts of anger and great sadness. Simple sentence structures and words were no longer within reach. It was as if the mind recognized their existence but the file was no longer readable, rendering what was once known completely inaccessible. A sense of frustration and helplessness began to present itself into every conversation. Even a simple conversation became fearful for her: *What if the person asked a familiar question, and I started to answer but could not finish?* Or, *the answer was so outrageous that I would give my struggle away.* The difficulty was not in the never knowing, but the knowing and failure to recall what should be readily available. So she would enter into dialogue assuming she could fully engage only to discover too late that she no longer had access to her acquired knowledge. Simple questions became frustrating, aggressive, and exhausting. *Why are you asking me that? You should know the answer. You are just trying to frustrate me.* In spite of these great difficulties, she would have moments of miraculous recovery as the Lord manifested the power of His spoken Word through Jeanette with articulate precision on several occasions. One particular moment took place less than a year before she finally succumbed to the disease.

We were lying in bed watching the news coverage of the Philippine typhoon in 2013.[32] It was named the Super Typhoon Haiyan because of the massive destruction it caused leaving 6,300 people dead, another 27,000 injured, and many more missing. By its destructive end, more than sixteen million people were affected with four million left homeless. I thought Jeanette was asleep. Suddenly she grabbed my arm and squeezed it to the point of pain. Without warning, she began passionately praying out loud under the anointing of the Holy Spirit. She spoke with authority and with ease even though for months she struggled to just complete a simple sentence. She described in detail the plight of those ravaged by the storm and flooding. She prayed for the victims, especially the children who had been separated from their parents, asking the Lord to reunite these families. She prayed for the wounded and those lost at

---

32 Meagan Singer, "2013 State of the Climate: Record-breaking Super Typhoon Haiyan," Climate.gov, July 13,2014, www.climate.gov, accessed 1/22/2016.

sea. I lay there mesmerized with this powerful witness of her prayers and passion. Surely this cannot be. She is incapable of speaking forth her heart and understanding the totality of the needs of these people. Yet she prayed on. She even prayed that donors would send large donations; she prayed for the relief workers and for the pastors who would have the terrible responsibilities of burying the dead. In this miraculous moment, I realized this was not just a personal prayer but a global intercession.

Jeanette, at that moment led by the Holy Spirit, lifted up before a Holy God the needs of a broken nation. What does all this mean? It means the disease can—in its great battle for the mind—take away cognition, causing our loved ones to be both physically and mentally handicapped, even close down many of their vital organs; but it cannot take captive their personal relationship with Jesus Christ. That is secured in the One, Eternal, Triune God. That relationship was well in place before Alzheimer's disease. As a beloved daughter of the living Abba Father, He wasn't done with her yet. On that day, it was His Spirit calling out of her the power of intercessory prayer for the sufferers in the Philippines. She ended the prayer with a long outburst of speaking in tongues. Then peacefully, almost suddenly, she went to sleep with no indication that she felt this was out of her ordinary daily walk with the Lord. Little did I know, as I witnessed this miraculous event, that she was slipping day by day into the final phase of her journey. Her doctor's initial pronouncement, two and a half years earlier, rang loud and clear in my heart: whatever you want to do with and for your wife, do it quickly. The next morning her speech impairments returned as if the previous night's prayer never occurred.

Aggressive and relentless in their conquest, the warrior plaques and tangles moved to the area where Jeanette's logic took place. An extreme left-brainer, Jeanette possessed extraordinary problem-solving and analytical skills. She was a strategist and had an uncanny ability to see how things fit together. As the disease progressed, what used to be natural and normal processes (balancing a checkbook or organizing a major event) became impossible tasks. When this was suddenly gone, the "natural" became extremely unnatural. It is what added to the language confusion. Her sentence structure and communication skills were disorganized and nonsensical. It was more than just a feeling of helplessness; she was grasping for a slippery sense of control as if she had her thoughts in hand but not a good handle or grasp on them. So they slipped through her fingers forever lost to the conquest occurring in her mind.

In a seemingly natural progression of an unnatural disease, that area of Jeanette's brain that controlled her moods, emotions, laughter, anger, and the correct expressions of grief was the next to be under siege. Having lost these coping disciplines, Jeanette would demonstrate that loss with an onslaught of odd behaviors and outbursts, confusion, distance, unwarranted fears, and most especially, the inability to know and communicate with those in her presence. In one instance we were sitting in a Sunday morning service. The pastor was preaching his heart out. Right in the middle of his most passionate point Jeanette yelled out, "You are a liar! That's not true. He's not telling the truth!" Maybe I too had become susceptible to the disease because instead of being ashamed—as many might be—I laughed in spite of our bizarre circumstance. It was funny. The poor pastor tried hard to recover his flow but failed. I doubt many saw the beauty or the humor of what occurred that day. Many may have secretly rebuked me for bringing her to church knowing her state of mind. Our services are meant to be perfect— stained glass perfect. All things in their proper place and everyone victorious over disease or mental deficiency. But that day the Lord chose our church to allow the body to really reflect His reach, His embrace. He decided that individuals who live with major impairments can be given a visible and necessary place at the Master's table. So, Jeanette made herself known, visible. Not locked away or hidden. Present, with us. And, for better or worse, us with her. Isn't that what we vow as we take membership with the body of Christ? A covenantal not contractual relationship. Was it awkward? Absolutely. Praise be to God. That awareness is what breaks us out of the shadows of what is real. It confronts our false and pretentious notions about *Koinonia*, that mystical fellowship only obtainable by the Spirit of the Living God. It reminds us that we are rich, poor, black, white, Hispanic, healthy, dysfunctional, recovered and sick. We are all these things collectively and communally. By His mercy, we are working it out, not according to our calculations, but by submission to His greater mission in this world and in us.

> *Jeanette made herself known, visible. Not locked away or hidden. Present, with us. And, for better or worse, us with her.*

As her condition worsened, we had to come up with our own battle plan in this war. She was no longer safe to make even her day to day decisions. Our initial task was to ensure Jeanette's care and safety as her cognitive abilities began to quickly deteriorate. It was obvious that we needed more support. Safety quickly became an issue. We brought our house up to the highest possible safety standards. Jeanette was beginning to wander, so we added dead bolts. As much as we tried, there were still occasions when she would find an unlocked door and let herself out. On two occasions this turned into a frantic search for her in our neighborhood. One of these incidents included the assistance of law-enforcement officers and neighbors.

In the evenings, shadows would play tricks on Jeanette's already exhausted mind, which seemed to add to her confusion. Thus, we added extra lighting to help reduce some of these growing symptoms. Other accommodations included moving the furniture around to allow her to safely and easily navigate from room to room and updating the bathroom. We needed Jeanette to be able to safely get in and out of the shower. Since a tub would require her to step over the sides and to sit in the bottom, we went to a standing shower with a shower seat and rails. Next, we contracted with a home care agency for approximately 10 hours per day to give the family additional support. On the recommendation of Jeanette's nutritionist, we developed a food plan that called for extra proteins, plenty of fruit, vegetables, and very lean meats. In spite of these changes, over a period of three years Jeanette went from 130 lbs. to 102 when she died in August 2014.

All great generals know they are only as strong as the network of allies they create. My next job was to ensure that we partnered with all the right people in the ways that would best connect our need with their specific skill set. Our three adult children and five grandchildren were our primary partners in this endeavor. Since we had agreed from the beginning that Jeanette would not be institutionalized, all of us had to adjust our schedules so that at least one family member was with her at all times. The kids were my "on-call" support. Each provided a vital and necessary role in her care and even my care. They provided much needed respites when the day-to-day duties were too much for me or when I was called out of town to tend to business. They did so with great distances between us and with small children in tow. They did this always with commitment and love for Jeanette and me. I am truly indebted to them for their care and many sacrifices. Without them Jeanette would not have been able to remain at home with me.

Not all of my partners were so generous with their care and commitments. Our experiences with the various medical support systems were, to say the least, mixed. Initially we chose a nationally recognized clinic for Jeanette's diagnostic review. They gave to us what I would call a medical "road map" for timely care and needs as Jeanette would progress through the various stages of Alzheimer's disease. But as the months rolled into the next year, we saw less and less of the doctors and more of administrators or nursing assistants. The clinic was so overloaded with clients that often we sat for hours waiting for someone to answer our list of questions concerning Jeanette's medicines, behavior, and our role in making sure we were on target with her home care. We came to realize that most medical doctors in this field spend little time with clients or their caregivers. They were functioning more as prescription managers and referral agents. Thankfully, we recognized very early in the process that the ball was in our court; we had to aggressively seek those who would give us the time and direction we needed. Consequently, we transferred Jeanette to another clinic with a doctor who saw her more regularly and whose personality seemed more suited to Jeanette.

This didn't resolve all our issues; Jeanette despised these clinic visits and was not shy about it. With her strong personality and stubbornness she could make the best of the medical personnel reactive rather than proactive. Trying to lead her, I decided to come up with a better strategy. First, prior to the visit, I prayed with Jeanette, gave her lots of hugs, talked very privately about the upcoming visit and its purpose, and reassured her of my constant presence. Second, I played music prior to leaving to put her in a more relaxed state. Third, I took lots of goodies, candy, or some other treat. Fourth, I left with plenty of time to spare so that I could drive slow and cautiously (the ride frightened her and made the visit even more threatening).

Finally, once we arrived at the doctor's office or clinic, I put her in an area with good lighting and used my cell phone to play some old hymns while gently speaking with her. All these strange surroundings frightened and confused her, and it was up to me and her other primary caregivers to try to neutralize the environment. Interestingly, her care experts didn't seem to take serious those external factors which could make the visit less frightening for all their patients suffering from Alzheimer's disease. This was just further proof of the vast difference between treating a disease and treating a person. On my end, I tried my best to personally get to know and partner with these medical specialists, even participating in their conferences.

On one occasion I was invited by Jeanette's doctor to speak at a medical conference with doctors, nurses, and other Alzheimer's care personnel. I told the audience that many of their clients, like Jeanette, had lived through the Great Depression, World War II, Vietnam, and so many other experiences. The lives of these individuals were necessary and important in the formation of all of our lives—young and old. I described for them my own experiences of caring for Jeanette's personal needs, like bathing and cleaning her up after her battle with uncontrollable bowels, and paralleled it to the job of Joseph of Arimathea and Nicodemus who prepared Jesus's broken and bloody body following His death on the cross (John 19: 38-42). I implored of them, "Caring for these, who represent the very best of all of us, is more than just a job. Like Joseph and Nicodemus's care of Christ's broken body, our care of these individuals is a sacred, unforgettable ritual, with heavenly consequences." The room was reverently silent. The leader of the conference, with tears in her eyes, approached the podium. After a short but careful pause, she instructed us to stand, join hands, and pray silently for those who treat Alzheimer's patients and those whose very existence

> *Like Joseph and Nicodemus's care of Christ's broken body, our care of these individuals is a sacred, unforgettable ritual, with heavenly consequences.*

depend on our personal touch and treatment. The experience of that moment for me was bigger than I could have imagined. I hadn't realized how much *I* needed to be heard and have my experience validated. I needed my anguish, my frustration, and my own sacred acts of care acknowledged. That day they became witnesses relativizing my own testimony as one touched and changed by Alzheimer's disease.

This and other sources assisted me as I continued to gather an army of support and allies. Thank God for the internet. Technology proved to be an invaluable weapon in our fight, connecting us to many of the front-line caregivers—those who provided around-the-clock care and those faced with the difficult decision to institutionalize their loved one. They were blatantly honest as they shared the good, the difficult, and the impossible. I plugged into their vast networks: Facebook, newsletters, national, regional and local associations, plus any other informal communication system that connected me with others in our situation. This informal network of allies and personal support systems surrounded and uplifted anyone who indicated they were struggling. This specialized force bombarded struggling hearts with an array of notes, articles, and personal calls. We were bound by our cause and our pain. Dependent on this growing community, we learned rather quickly that in caring for Jeanette we needed both medical specialists and the "boots on the ground" caregivers or formal in-home care.

For two long years home care assistants provided a necessary service to our family. As much as we wanted to, we simply were not equipped to provide the extensive care she needed on our own.

Jeanette was never excluded from planning the care process; her opinions were always heard even when they became disjointed or nonsensical. She would make statements like: "You know you are not telling the truth," or "Who are you to tell me what to do? Shut up. You do not know what you are talking about." In this progressed stage of the disease, she at times became verbally hostile. We learned that if we waited a little while she would change and become pleasant again. However, for those with long hair, beware. Jeanette, in her most severe state, would grab hair and hold on for dear life. This is why our in-home assistants were so vital. The caregivers helped with all the various duties in caring for Jeanette: bathing, dressing, safety, continence, eating, and other daily tasks we take for granted. These 15-20 care givers were essential and several of them were exceptional.

Some of our best experiences with these dedicated caregivers occurred as a result of us humanizing one another. We shared our stories and our trust—my trust of them with Jeanette and theirs of me to guide them in caring for Jeanette. This kind of mutual care allowed for open dialogue and teaching to occur intentionally, yet organically. They taught me their craft through various techniques and practices; I taught them how to personalize their craft by being interested in the lives and stories of the ones they care for (recipients and their families).

All of our outside caregivers came with their own financial, social, and spiritual needs. Some of our best spiritual experiences during this time came with unplanned prayer and worship with our in-home care team. A couple of these caregivers gave their hearts to the Lord in our home. I must admit that, in the beginning, this new role and calling seemed so insignificant to me. My how the Lord has a way of showing us that His plans are bigger than our ability (sometimes willingness) to see them. Maybe the battle we think we are fighting (and losing) is not the battle we are truly engaged in. These women were a part of His plan, His battle plan. While Jeanette seemed to be losing a battle for her mind and life, we were really winning a battle for hearts. A plan that was for Jeanette's benefit *and for their benefit.*

In addition to our many assistants, the Lord sent many visitors: friends, colleagues, family, and curious acquaintances. For the most part, this was a vital source of support and encouragement to us both. However, not every visit brought strength. Sometimes these visits wore us down with unnecessary tension and conflict. Unfortunately for caregivers, this can often be the case. Those outside of the primary care team are often uninformed and come with preconceived notions about what should or should not be done on behalf of the one suffering from Alzheimer's disease. Although well-meaning in their efforts, their visits are unproductive and taxing on those of us who are already exhausted from a demanding care process.

Belonging to such a large, close-knit family, it was difficult to keep all of Jeanette's family well-informed and understanding of her developing mental state. These visits with her three brothers and two sisters were, for the most part, pleasant and meaningful. As Jeanette worsened she became more and more reluctant and less interested in their childhood stories. Watchfully yet cautiously, I affirmed the benefits of these visits while ensuring that those who visited her took into consideration not only who she was, but who she was becoming as a result of damaged brain cells. Some were quick learners. Others, like me, tried desperately to resurrect the old Jeanette—even to the very end. Their unwillingness to learn and hear God speak in the midst of her painful struggles and ours cost them the opportunity to be cleansed by the crisis—a lesson he was beginning to unfold in my spirit.

Thankfully, we did not have a lot of challenging visits. Most of our visits were timely and welcomed, like Jeanette's last visit with her older brother John, and his wife Camille. Growing up, Jeanette and John were like grits and gravy; where you saw one, you saw the other. Yet over time they had grown somewhat apart. Maybe that is why this visit was so meaningful to us. The gap that had formed between them was not present that day, the Lord was. They hugged each other and talked like the two of them had done so many years earlier. Then as John and Camille were leaving, Jeanette reached out and began to pray for John. With her hands on the head of her beloved brother, she blessed him in the name of the Lord.

Unexpectedly, a great outpouring of God's wonderful Holy Spirit fell upon that room. Her prayer was more than just a prayer for safe travels; it was a blessing likened to those biblical patriarchs who spoke blessings over their children before dying. The blessing itself was a type of inheritance. In that final prayer, she extended to him a legacy of faith and covering that can only be satisfied by the Lord God, himself. It was her gift and her good bye. Although it was their last visit together before her death, it is one that will carry over into

Paradise when they are once again joined for all eternity with the entire family of God.

So many family members, friends, and chaplains visited to extend their love, prayers and appreciation for our ministry. In a crisis of this magnitude, these are the people we must surround ourselves with if we are going to survive. They were the arsenal of friends and loved ones who faithfully prayed, called, followed up, dialogued, and chose to be present in the difficult, even darkest hours. These co-journeyers were a constant reminder that we were never alone. We battled with a great band of brothers and sisters who faithfully made themselves available to carry burdens that were often too great to bear alone. This is what true *koinonia* looks like, not the stained-glassed Sunday morning version. Real *koinonia* inter-twines our lives with others who understand and have the shared experience of our Lord's love, His comfort and gentleness, and the blessed knowledge that because we belong to Him we belong to one another. Therefore, *koinonia* incites all of us to be first responders. To not run from a messy war scene or worse, turn the channel, but to ready ourselves to be the care others need. That is what these many friends and family members provided for us—the simplicity and power of *koinonia*.

> *Koinonia incites all of us to be first responders. To not run from a messy war scene or worse, turn the channel, but to ready ourselves to be the care others need.*

In spite of our great efforts to fight back, the war inside her continued to make its advancements. The last onslaught of attacks, the *blitzkreig* if you will, were the last great battles of her cognitive person. She lost her sense of taste and smell. Food had become neutral, bland. Eating was reduced to a task that she would forget if we hadn't provided the meals ourselves. Next she lost the memory of her life and history. I felt it was my job to keep them alive when possible. Having been married for so long, I knew all her favorite stories about our life together. This was a very special time of remaining connected with Jeanette. However, this may have been the most painful to witness. Jeanette would wander throughout the house, trying intensively to figure out each picture on the wall or peer out the window like a prisoner dreaming of the opportunity to escape. For five years we worked hard to keep alive all those stories of her life as a child with a Mom and Dad she adored. Sometimes I would tease her by asking, "Who do you love the most, me or your Mom and Dad?" To avoid my entrapment, she would always respond, "That is for me to know and you to figure out." Eventually the days arrived when, like a nightmare out of the blue, the strong images of her dad and mom began to fade. Aware of this fading, she became more frightened than I had ever seen her. She would pace the floor calling for them, begging for someone to help her find them. Finally, she would wear herself out with this anguish, sit down, and weep uncontrollably. I would try to ease the pain by telling her how her precious parents had died many years earlier and were enjoying their heavenly rest, but my words could bring no comfort to her ailing heart. She would reply, "Yes, I know that, but do they not know how much I need to see and touch them right now?" Within just a few short months even this grief of their absence would disappear and she would never again mention their names or her many wonderful memories of her time with them. As time continued, she not only lost the memories of her past, she no longer could recall her present family. Our marriage of sixty-six years had no meaning; her three children and five grandchildren were lost to her. Finally, Jeanette had difficulty with balance, often falling when trying to stand up. Soon she would become mostly bed-bound.

Battle Lost. Cognitive Faculties Captive.

Through the eyes of her daughter:

Mom always prepared a perfect holiday gathering for us. Thanksgiving 2011 was anything but that for me. That was the day the painful reality of her life—our lives—set in for me permanently. That morning was pleasant. Mom let me fix her hair and help her get dressed. It seemed it was going to be a good day, as good as it could be under these circumstances. At this point it was a struggle to get Mom out of the house; every change in her routine upset her greatly. So, having dinner at Dale's inherently posed some threat to her day. As Dad and I got Mom into the car and drove Mom down to Dale's house, I was optimistic this was going to be a fun family gathering. By that time, any semblance we had of a traditional family gathering was a treasure to each of us. As we got Mom out of the car and walked up to the house, Dad whispered to me, "Your mom asked me who that nice lady was (referring to me)." This was the time I had been dreading. I was no longer her daughter, just a nice lady who helped her out. We got into the house and sat at the table. As Dad prayed our Thanksgiving prayer, the tears welled up in my eyes and began to pour. The realization that I was no longer her daughter hit me like a brick wall. I could not contain my grief. I excused myself to the bathroom and fought to stop the tears. Unable to contain them, I cried uncontrollably. I don't know how long I was in the bathroom, eventually my sister-in-law came in and sat with me. She understood the grief. I knew things would never be the same. Somehow I mustered enough courage to return to the meal, but this Thanksgiving was, by far, the hardest ever. I knew that, although my mother did not know me as her daughter, I would have to figure out a new way to relate to her. I would have to respect her and not force my needs on her, but respect the world as she saw it.

The grieving would continue for some time to come. In a sense, this was the first grief—losing her emotionally; the second would come in her physical death.

New Names to Fit New Perceptions

The loss of memory forced Jeanette to re-name persons around her to fit her new reality. It was up to us (family, caregivers, and friends) to reject or accept her new reality as part of ours. Without really understanding all these changes in her behavior, Jeanette began to see me as her husband and companion, as well as many other roles. My identification ranged during her long ordeal from "Bob" her husband to "Papa" her grandfather to "Mr. Boss Man" and "Pastor." I was many things to Jeanette but rarely her husband. "Bob," her husband, was often missing in her mind. In fact, she would often make excuses for this "missing Bob." I had become a phantom to her. I was fully visible and present but no longer seen by her. Yet in her searching for me, I believe she drew me nearer to her by attaching these other personalities to me. It was the only way both of us could keep each other visible and immersed in one another's lives.... .

Bob's Father. As much as I loved my father, this title did not measure up in her eyes to that of her grandfather. Once, with a frightened look on her face, she stated that she wanted a very private meeting with me. We went into an upstairs room for privacy. She stated in a quiet tone, as if she did not want anyone else to hear her words, "I need to tell you that your dad touched me in a very inappropriate manner. You need to get him out of our house or I will leave this place!"

Without trying to convince her that I was the one who touched her, I simply responded, "He will leave immediately." I learned quickly to respond in the manner she expected. I didn't argue with her or try to convince her of the truth; I affirmed her fears and need. More than anything I wanted to assure that she was safe and that I would never let anyone harm her. So I *kicked him out* without a second thought. Remember, perception was always reality.

Mr. Boss Man. Because I was the general manager of her care, instructing caregivers and family members who came to assist me, she would jokingly say, "Who died and left you in charge?" She couldn't possibly understand all that was being done on her behalf. So, her witty comments and sarcasm was always met with laughter and an extra hug which she readily resisted. (I was the hired hand and had no business hugging her.) She had a great way about her even in these progressed states of dementia. Her strong, brilliant personality and witty sense of humor is what had always drawn me to her. Thankfully, the best parts of her still remained even in that new land and new reality. Yes, the whole of it was very, very hard. Yet joy and laughter was often present. It was that enduring joy of the Lord that allowed us to find the humor in even our most bizarre predicaments. Besides, I was just thankful that I was allowed to be anyone to her—whoever she needed me to be—as long as she allowed me to return to her daily.

> *I was just thankful that I was allowed to be anyone to her—whoever she needed me to be—as long as she allowed me to return to her daily.*

Pastor. In spite of her developing Alzheimer's condition, Jeanette continued to demonstrate a deep spiritual relationship with the Lord. A few times during the week we had a short fifteen minute worship service. Sometimes our contracted caregivers joined in with us. Initially, she would lead us in an old hymn but that soon passed. She never lost the ability to pray though. Even though at intervals she was confused about who I was and what my relationship was with her, she and I would pray together for long periods of time. Her prayers were full of passion and zeal for the Lord. While words and phrases were disjointed and seemingly illogical, I knew the Lord understood every bit of what she wanted to communicate to Him. In these times the Holy Spirit's presence was wonderfully felt. Time and again, Jeanette would raise her bony hands and speak in a heavenly language as the Spirit would lead. No matter how advanced the disease, she never seemed to lose touch with her life-long relationship with the Lord. She loved Him and loved to lift up her prayers to Him. She miraculously maintained this practice until about three days before she died. Her example of faith and commitment fed my soul on those difficult days, days when I felt a vast gulf between God and me. An example that continued beyond her death.

Papa. In the later stages of this disease, she finally gave me the distinct title of "Papa," the name of her grandfather whom she dearly loved as a child. Jeanette had seen her papa as a pivotal player in her early developmental years. Even though he died in 1942, she, in her need to capture something sacred out of her past, chose this name for me. I was honored to be an "image" of a person she deeply loved growing up in Kettle Island, KY. Often I would find her walking around calling for me, "Papa! Papa! Where are you?" This may have been one of my favorite roles. Mostly because he was such a beloved part of her life and history. He would often surprise her with special gifts.

On her fourth birthday, he asked her to dance the "Charleston" as a prerequisite for her birthday gift, a little red rocker. One day she relived this event for us in our living room. She danced jubilantly. She danced as if she were a child again. She danced with great pride in spite of her aging limitations. To me, she was breathtaking—just as she had always been. For the grandkids, she was magical. They loved seeing Oma so childlike and free to experience these past events anew. They smiled and cheered for her, hugging her with delight after her big production.

Unnamed Roles. Keeping Jeanette occupied required more than rehearsing her life story. I would often entertain her in an attempt to divert her attention from the more invasive roles. I chose this role as an attempt to stay attached to her as long as I could. It wasn't a role she gave or assigned to me. It was a role I wanted. I would make up little playful lyrics and sing to her. Generally, I would tease her like an older child to a younger child. She seemed to love it; sometimes she would even clap and hug me with a big smile after one of my shenanigans. But this role—this distraction—could only last temporarily. As my role became more intrusive to her, she saw me more as a violator than a helper. These feelings came during the times when I had to clean her up after an explosive bowel movement or had to give her a bath. If I had a female worker in the bathroom with me she would tolerate my presence much better. But alone in this exposed state? That was very difficult for her. It tapped into her long history of modesty. She was sometimes terrified of me, like I was a violator of her most sacred dignity.

These were moments when our realities could not exist side-by-side. In fact, their intersecting paths collided in these moments. I did all I could do to deal with this *misidentification*. To say that it was painful is a gross understatement. I loved her and would never do harm to her. My heart was profoundly wounded by the thought that she lost a sense of our long and loving relationship. I tried to find comfort in knowing that she was incapable of understanding, but even knowledge could not remove the realities of her hostile rejections. I even pleaded with her that the experience was difficult for both of us, to please let me finish cleaning her up so we could just be done. For the most part, we simply survived the experience. Relieved it was over and she was cleaned up, I would bring her tea and cookies. Then, worn out, I would sit down beside her and turn on some music to comfort both of us. Afterwards she would often touch my heart with her kind words of gratitude, "I know you work so hard, and I know you care for me." Her words were as a healing balm following what were often some of the most cutting experiences of caring for her. It had to be the Lord who shifted her from that jarring response of fear to that gentle response of gratitude. Though mere words, they satisfied my desire to remain connected and mended my broken-spirit.

In those most difficult nights, I realized how similar our realities were. Like Jeanette, I too felt detached, alone, even fearful. Jeanette, my wife, the mother of our children, and my long-term ministry colleague had disappeared. I now had to deal with her many personalities. I would think to myself, "This woman who has been married to me for 65 years, raised and nurtured our kids, spent long hours praying for me while I was in combat or other difficult military assignment, and my ministry partner wherever the Lord assigned us, now does not even know who I am!"

That Jeanette, it seemed, was gone forever. As I reflect back on those feelings I realize that I grieved deeply and had to come to terms with two significant losses. The first loss was the Jeanette who

I knew and experienced before the onslaught of Alzheimer's; the second loss was the Jeanette she became as the disease developed over a period of several years. Both of these persons, the former and the latter which left her in a "childlike state" were deeply attached to my soul. And both of these losses had their own characteristics which had to be dealt with separately. Without a doubt, my wife left an everlasting mark on my life. There was never a moment that I didn't love her. We were one…by choice and by divine design. Yet the latter Jeanette, the most vulnerable Jeanette, bound herself to me in a most unique and permanent way. While our need for each other never changed, we experienced it in very different ways. She needed me to provide protection, care, shelter, and other basic needs. I needed her to allow me to remain a necessary figure in our story, to live as close to her new land as possible. When her journey took her beyond my ability as a travel companion, I found myself still waiting for her to find her way back to me. I know it was irrational, but my mind and soul was still bound to her by a vow I made over 60 years earlier…for better or for worse…in sickness or in health…until death do us part…*she was my home.* No matter which Jeanette I had, there was *no place like home.*

Who Am I?[33]

Who am I? They often tell me
I stepped from my cell's confinement
Calmly, cheerfully, firmly
Like a Squire from his country house.

Who am I? They often tell me
I used to speak to my wardens
Freely and friendly and clearly,
As though I were mine to command.

Who am I? They also tell me
I bore the days of misfortune
Equably, smilingly, proudly
Like one accustomed to win

Am I then really that which other men tell of?
Or am I only what I myself know of myself?
Restless and longing and sick, like a bird in a cage.
Struggling for breath, as though hands were compressing my throat.
Yearning for colors, for flowers, for the voices of birds.
Thirsting for words of kindness, for neighborliness.
Tossing in expectations of great events.

---

33   Deitrich Bonhoeffer, "Who Am I?" International Bonhoeffer Society English Language Section, 1945, November 11, 2015, www.dbonhoeffer. org/who-was-db2.htm.

Powerlessly trembling for friends at an infinite distance.
Weary and empty at praying, at thinking, at making.
Faint and ready to say farewell to it all

Who am I? This or the Other?
Am I one person today and tomorrow another?
Am I both at once? A hypocrite before others.
And before myself a contemptible woebegone weakling?
Or is something within me still like a beaten army
Fleeing in disorder from victory already achieved?

Who am I? They mock me, these lonely questions of mine.
Whoever I am, Thou knowest, O God, I am thine!

Deitrich Boenhoffer, 1945, Flossian concentration camp

Chapter 8

Paradise Found: What Will Remain When All Seems Lost?

The Final Phase

"The Lord turned to [Gideon] and said,
"Go in the strength you have and save Israel out of Midian's hand.
Am I not sending you?"
Judges 6:14 (NIV)

Paradise Lost

This final phase of Alzheimer's came to us initially as a "Paradise Lost." It was the culmination of everything the disease sought to strip from her: her memories, her story, her ability to communicate and effectively express emotions, her intellect and reason, and so much more. Much of Jeanette's acquired knowledge was erased and her strongly developed personality and independent spirit was quickly fading. No one gets a free pass with Alzheimer's. Every phase must make its presence known, starting slow then picking up its destructive momentum until finally an inevitable death.

By all medical standards, the *old Jeanette* was gone and the new, often agitated, child-like Jeanette had taken up residence in the *old Jeanette's* body. She was intermittently both adult and child. At times it seemed that these two were in competition with each other. One or the other would appear unannounced and move off the scene as quickly as she arrived. She was like a child housed in an adult body which, under the right conditions, would rise up strongly, with frustration, agitation, even anger over simple tasks that had become impossible, like getting up from a chair or responding to a question. With these physical changes came a state of hopelessness. In those moments, neither seemed present. She seemed lost, disconnected, maybe even estranged. She seemed to be asking herself, *Who are these people? Why are they telling me things that do not factor in my core feelings? What are all these strange objects?* And, *why do they continue to claim these objects are mine when I know they are not?'*

As bad as the tangible forgetting was, it could not compare to the *unseen forgetting:* the slow deterioration of her vital organs. It was as if her brain had been hijacked and was no longer able to communicate with her vital organs, and so they began to malfunction. They

> *No one gets a free pass with Alzheimer's.*

178

could no longer carry out their task of keeping her alive. We were no longer dealing with "minor" issues. From this point until her death, they were all major. Her kidneys and bowels began to malfunction; she had difficulty standing; she experienced anxiety attacks; not to mention, a number of secondary physical problems, including bowel blockage and diarrhea. These many physical changes left her in a state of helplessness. We found ourselves running from one doctor to another, and, on a few occasions, to our local emergency room.

She wasn't the only one feeling helpless. The path through this new land seemed to be leading us far outside of *our* paradise. The terrain was fierce and the experience harsh. In our desire to remain with her, our hearts cried out, "Regardless of the complexities of this long journey, let it continue. Let us keep her in whatever state *You* put her in for just a few more days, months, or even years." My cry was not in denial; we were too far into this journey to deny the inevitable. I knew the Lord was going to finally bring this journey to its end. Selfishly, I wanted her to remain; I was still bound to her even though I could feel the ripping of her soul from mine as she moved closer to eternity and further from me. We were one and I didn't know how to be me without her. So we waited fearfully, anxiously. Truly, like Gideon, I wanted to hide in a winepress from this relentlessly brutal intruder. In my weariness, I wanted my opportunity, my face-to-face, to ask the Lord:

"…if the Lord is with us, why has all this happened to us? Where are all His wonders that our ancestors told us about when they said,

'Did not the Lord bring us up out of Egypt?' But now the Lord has abandoned us and put us into the hand of Midian."[34]

So apparent in Gideon's questioning was his love for his people, frustration over his own plight and fear for their shared future, but most of all, for God to be the God he *wanted* Him to be. He was looking for God to be the Deliverer God and not the "*with us in our struggle*" God. I too despaired out of my great love for her and our children, who were experiencing this grief with me. I too was exhausted and frustrated over her situation, *our situation*, and feared the inevitable end that would come from the perils of this final phase. But most of all, I wanted God to deliver us—her—from this dreadful disease even though I knew that God was *with us* as we walked this path. It didn't seem fair for her to experience such torment when she had been so faithful all those years in her walk with the Lord. What would be left to demonstrate the basic core values of her long walk with a faithful Lord after Alzheimer's disease finishes its task? In *my version* of fair, it didn't add up. *What is fair or compassionate in that? What would we be left of Jeanette that we could still hold onto and celebrate?*

The questions themselves were my "Midian-like giants" to fight. Yet even in my despair, I could sense the Lord responding mercifully to me from my own text of accusation. "The Lord turned to him and said, 'Go in **the strength you have** and save Israel out of Midian's hand. Am I not sending you?'"[35] What I love about this response is

---

34   Jud. 6:13 NIV

35   Jud. 6:16 NIV [Emphasis added]

that it didn't begin with words but with an alignment between man and deity. The Lord turned *toward* Gideon. He made it clear where the focus of this conversation was. Not on circumstances, not on a better pedigree, not on an emotionally charged, puffed-up motivational speech that can't deliver in the real world; His attention was on Gideon, the recipient of his commission. His *turning toward* was an intimate act of looking Gideon in the eye and seeing him, acknowledging exactly where he was circumstantially, physically, spiritually, and emotionally. It was an intentional move from the Holy Other God to the Ever Present, With Us God. His "turning to" was a direct answer to Gideon's searching, *where is God, and why has He abandoned us?* His words reveal a great desire on his part for God to return to him and his people. So the Lord God of Israel appeared and turned His attention to Gideon. In my despairing, my fearful, hiding place, the God of Paradise heard my cry and came to me. The God of the Angel Armies turned His attention toward me in my searching. In His gaze I could sense the Spirit responding, "Quit asking why this happened. Focus on what *remains.*" In other words, "Go in the strength *you already have!*" That strength of Spirit found in the everlasting [mutual] love of God from which nothing can separate us. Just as Jeanette loved Him with a supernatural love, so too did I. I have loved my God faithfully in the everlasting love that He cultivated in the very core of my spirit. Just as her obvious love of God remained, so my love for Him remained, and the Lord was declaring it to be my strength. In other words, my strength was found two-fold: first, in an everlasting covenantal relationship with the Almighty God; and second, in the witnessing of Jeanette's continued and expressed, unfailing love of her Lord and Savior, Jesus Christ—even in a state of progressed dementia.

The Psalmist[36] said it like this: "I love you [fervently and devotedly], O LORD, my strength." Like the psalmist, I knew the Lord to be our rock, our fortress, deliverer, trusted strength, our buckler, the horn of our salvation, and high tower (Ps. 18:2 KJV). While witnessing the ever increasing deterioration of her frail body, I could sense the "sorrows of death" all around me (Ps. 18:4). So, I cried out to the Lord and he heard my voice. "He bowed the heavens also and came down" (Ps. 18:9). He *turned to* me and lit a candle in my darkness (Ps. 18:28). He encircled me with strength and made my way blameless, making "my feet like hinds' feet [able to stand firmly and tread safely on paths of testing and trouble]" (Ps. 18:33 AMP).

In that moment of alignment, I could see more clearly not just the source of my strength, but the strength which remained and presented itself daily in her life and in mine. You see, again the issue of perspective arose. Some see Gideon hiding in a vat from his enemy, but God saw a survivor willing to strategize and improvise in the midst of life threatening conditions. God was naming me according to who I had always been, not who I felt like I had become. Jeanette and I were not impoverished of strength; we were survivors who knew how to thrive in seasons of famine and devastation. Just as Paul declared in Philippians chapter four, I had learned how to be sustained in all circumstances—on empty or with plenty. For it is God—alone—who gives me (us) the

---

36 Ps. 18:9 AMP

strength to endure all things. The candle He lit in my darkness was this: Alzheimer's disease is a powerful force that would ultimately destroy Jeanette's physical body and mind because the physical man was meant to wear out. It is finite. But salvation is of the Lord; it lasts—or remains—forever (Is. 51:6)! Alzheimer's disease could take her body, but it could not detach Jeanette from her great love of God. It is the strength that remained and would ultimately carry her home.

The strength which enabled us to endure this season wasn't just her faithful love of God, but my witness of it. He was calling me in that moment to embrace what could not be destroyed by this world: her deep love for her Lord, Jesus Christ, of which I was a privileged witness. Daily, I watched her remain true to values which were deeply ingrained in her heart while unable to even designate them as valuable. The retention of these morals was a testament that neither nature nor any other worldly force can remove from us our Belovedness. It is that identity which separates believers, like Jeanette, from other Alzheimer's disease journeys. That uniqueness has at its core certain characteristics that cannot be totally destroyed by the disease. For Jeanette and other believers, this fortified characteristic is what some call a "moral personhood."[37] The idea that identity is centered much deeper in us than merely our memories.

Gideon had no memory of himself as a triumphant warrior; his family was part of the smallest clan. He was simply a farmer who

---

37 Alison Gopnik, "Is our Identity in Intellect, Memory or Moral Character?" The Wall Street Journal, Sept. 9, 2015, accessed November 21, 2015, http://www.wsj.com/articles/is-our-identity-in-intellect-memory-or-moral-character-1441812784.

was determined to thrive in the face of great oppression. That day, that face-to-face with the Almighty God forced a greater question into the picture than Gideon's need to reconcile the God he knew of and the *abandoning God* he believed he was experiencing. The real issue wasn't God's identity; it was Gideon's. For me, in her frailty, the question I was really searching an answer for wasn't who was God going to be in this last phase: the Deliverer God or the "With Us" God. I knew that He would be *both*. The real searching I was after, the search that the Lord needed to align me with, was *who is this new, frail Jeanette?* After everything was stripped away, what will remain of *her*? A few years ago, I came across a lesson put out by the para-church organization, Youth for Christ. In the lesson the author asked the participants to create a collage that would describe who they are. After several students shared their descriptions, they were asked to remove all of the pictures, word art, etc. from the page. The follow-up question was this: *If everything that describes you (parent, child, supervisor, laborer, intelligent, athletic, etc.) is taken away like those images, who would remain?* Wow, right? That is a powerful and poignant activity that really drives home the identity question, especially as Christians. I feared the answer to this as I saw her page empty out. The question of God's presence and our ability to endure this last phase was settled; what I was confronted with was naming what remained.

Who has the last word on identification? Is it the medical world, whose definition fits very well into that public face of Alzheimer's disease? This identification, however, is limited to those series of events which would lead to the eventual death of Jeanette. That

Jeanette shares a common citizenship with the millions around the world in the *land and language of Alzheimer's*. Their lives, behaviors, and emotional states are very similar, whether black, white, Asian, Hispanic, male, female, from the northern hemisphere or the southern. But the "private Jeanette" has developed certain patterns based on her long life in serving her family and her Lord. These patterns formed what we might call her "spiritual profile." In other words, is the "real Jeanette" that Jeanette which is the *result* of the disease or could her identity be centered much deeper into the very core of her soul? If so, is it that identity which really names her, not this other, more public identity?

According to columnist Alison Gopnik,[38] "Neurodegenerative diseases like Alzheimer's make especially vivid a profound question about human nature. In the tangle of neural connections that make up our brain, where am I?" and as these connections begin to unravel, "What happens to the person?" According to the social sciences, identity is derived from three sources: our experiences over the course of a lifetime, the culture we live in, and our DNA. Yet, as I looked upon that shell of Jeanette and listened to others describe this process as a stripping of her self-knowledge, I believed there was still more to her. I saw her recover her fullest self with clarity in moments of prophecy and prayer, then return to her shell. I knew that she wasn't completely gone, but had no words or understanding to conceptualize what I saw. Then, in the searching, God showed

---

38 Alison Gopnik, "Is our Identity in Intellect, Memory or Moral Character?" The Wall Street Journal, Sept. 9, 2015, accessed November 21, 2015, http://www.wsj.com/articles/is-our-identity-in-intellect-memory-or-moral-character-1441812784.

me a path toward understanding. Mildred Wynkoop,[39] author and theologian, writes in response to that age-old identity assessment:

*Much that he is he derives from his heritage, from his culture, from his relatedness with the total present, **but he is not locked hopelessly in this "prison."** In ways that baffle philosophy and science, man can and does elect to make contrary choices and thereby becomes a "new man." Jesus spoke to whatever it is about man that takes positions about "ultimate concerns"; and man's condemnation or approval, in God's sight, depended on what man did at this point.*

In other words, philosophy and the social sciences have decided that our personhood is formed in the images of this world, externally and internally; BUT, GOD has another opinion on the subject. Contrary to scientific evaluation, we are not locked into that "prison." What remained in Jeanette after everything was said and done was the likeness of her eternal, Creator God, the Imago Dei. Jeanette had decided a long time ago that this world would not be the Master Potter forming her in some image likened to this world. Rather, cultivated over a life span of love and commitment to the restoration of His image in her heart, she decided to align her personhood with Christ Jesus, the eternal and manifest Word

---

39 Mildred Bangs Wynkoop, (1972). A Theology of Love: the dynamic of Wesleyanism (Kansas City, Missouri: Beacon Hill Press of Kansas City, 1972), 167. [Emphasis added.]

of God, thereby choosing to be something better than this world could offer. Therefore, what remained—her faithful relatedness to God as beloved child—remained because it transcended this physical world, and nothing could distort or destroy her truest self, her moral personhood, imaged in the likeness of the Eternal God.

New studies give credibility to what Jeanette revealed and our family witnessed. According to a study by psychologist Nina Strohminger and philosopher Shaun Nichols,[40] our identity doesn't just come from a composite of memories; rather, it comes more from our moral character. These researchers challenged the argument that many philosophers and medical personnel have assumed for years: our identity is rooted in our accumulated knowledge.[41] By this standard, our truest self is gone when our accumulated knowledge and skills are gone. Little room is left for the moral self; yet isn't that exactly how we identify people?

> *Jeanette had decided a long time ago that this world would not be the Master Potter forming her in some image likened to this world. Rather, she decided to align her personhood with Christ Jesus, the eternal and manifest Word of God.*

40 Nina Strohminger and Shaun Nichols, "The Essential Moral Self. Psychological Science," Cognition, 131 (2014) 159-171, accessed November 21, 2015, www.elsevier.com/locate/COGNIT.

41 Alison Gopnik, "Is our Identity in Intellect, Memory or Moral Character?" The Wall Street Journal, Sept. 9, 2015, accessed November 21, 2015, http://www.wsj.com/articles/is-our-identity-in-intellect-memory-or-moral-character-1441812784.

They (we) are known by their gentleness, compassion, generosity, or the absence of these traits. These are the characteristics which either alienate us or connect us to the people around us. The capacity in which we are re-identified as holy, sanctified children of God is in direct correlation with our willingness to live that out in our human relationships.[42] "It's the part of us that goes beyond our own tangle of neurons to touch the brains and lives of others." Why? "Because the moral character is central to who we are... ."[43]

The study doesn't discredit the impact of memory or other historically validated influencers; rather, it simply gives spiritual formation its rightful place in the discussion. From the beginning, Adam and Eve, in their relationship with their Creator, were more than the sum parts of their human endeavors (their stories and memory of them). What gave validity and meaning to their life came from the Breath which breathed them into existence and the God who formed them with His own hands. They were created to share in the divine nature of their Creator God, Yahweh. The fact that this God claimed them, regardless of their later misbehavior, was that "X" factor which was demonstrated in Jeanette's battle with this deadly disease in so many different ways. She got angry and frustrated; she struggled with nurses and caregivers. She

---

42 Mildred Bangs Wynkoop, (1972). A Theology of Love: the dynamic of Wesleyanism (Kansas City, Missouri: Beacon Hill Press of Kansas City, 1972), chapter nine.

43 Alison Gopnik, "Is our Identity in Intellect, Memory or Moral Character?" The Wall Street Journal, Sept. 9, 2015, accessed November 21, 2015, http://www.wsj.com/articles/is-our-identity-in-intellect-memory-or-moral-character-1441812784.

had human moments, but never strayed from her moral foundations. She was so much more than the public Jeanette,[44] both in the initial stages, and certainly in these final stages. The deep moral and spiritual characteristics of Jeanette remained long after Alzheimer's had taken away "the public characteristics" of the disease. Being a Christian who depends on the Word of God and the presence of the Holy Spirit, I know there will always be that which can be "seen with the naked eye," and that which can only be "seen with spiritual eyes." This is a basic principle that makes the intersection of creation and salvation so interesting and inspiring. On the outside, humanity is frail and finite and imperfect; on the inside, those who choose the perfect to impact the imperfect are reborn and made a new creature. One, through a restorative relationship with Christ, is given a new identity of eternal nature in Christ. It is this transformation which allowed Jeanette—child of God—to remain; and it is what remains in us when we allow for Christ to make us His own too. For, "God and no one else gives us our deepest and enduring values. That is, unless we serve some 'idol' such as success, power, sex, money, drugs, etc."[45]

I know this to be true from witnessing Jeanette's journey. Regardless of the many cognitive impairments that came as a result of Alzheimer's disease, her deep, long-term traditional relationship with her Lord remained. It was the Lord who showed me this; I

---

44 See the Preface for more information on the Public and Private Faces of Alzheimer's disease.

45 Steven Land. Interviewed by Robert Crick. Personal interview. Cleveland, TN, November 2015.

wasn't able to see this on my own. Yes, I knew she had faithfully served Him from early childhood to her recent death. During those years, she was fully committed to Christian principles and practices. In living with her for sixty-six years, I never heard her utter a curse word, or for that matter even a slang word. Yet it was He who opened the eyes of my heart to see that even in her most agitated Alzheimer's state, she would get angry, but never use inappropriate language. In faith, it simply wasn't who she had decided she would be. Even when she would get disoriented or disturbed, she would come back to a quieter, more manageable disposition after given a few moments to quiet herself.

Her character wasn't the only remaining evidence of her personhood; her motherly nature and deep love of God remained. Even when she could not put words to her concerns and care for our children and our "spiritual children (chaplains)," Jeanette steadfastly and intuitively cared for them. Not in motherly advice or in those traditional ways we might identify motherhood. That wasn't a real possibility for her anymore. Rather, she mothered them through her intuitive care in prayer. Jeanette was my prayer warrior. She was the one that prayed me into an altar three months after we were married. Her deep sensitivity to those in need would drive her to persistent prayer until change occurred. She was not one of those persons who called on the Lord only when there was a crisis. Instead, it was her daily prayerful walk with the Lord that made the difference from my perspective. Sometimes I would jokingly tell her that she had insider knowledge with the Lord that gave her a one up on the rest of us. She was sensitive to the Spirit's leading and would often feel compelled to enter into prayer for one of our children or the chaplains under our care. Of course, as she advanced into the later stages of Alzheimer's, her prayers were often disorganized and difficult to follow. Yet a profound sense of God's presence and power was felt. Read carefully these recorded prayers (without editing) well into the last phases of her long battle with Alzheimer's.

In this excerpt, Jeanette prayed for Jonne, our daughter, as she was getting ready to return home after her holiday visit. Intertwined in the jumbled words is a recurring theme of motherly protection often sustained with images of motherly care. The emphasis on God's presence in her life undergirds her desire as a mom for her child to remain safely in the care of a trustworthy God. Likewise, the images of baths, good meals, health, and wisdom all reinforce her intuitive need to fulfill her duties as Mom. This prayer isn't just a nice good-bye prayer; it is further evidence of that created identity—reflective of our Abba Father—which never releases us to be anything other than He creates us to be.

Christmas Day, 2013

Father, in the name of Jesus, we ask that the presence of God Almighty would be poured out on Jonne today as she leaves here to go home. And Father, you know these are not just want to's, rather, things that the Lord wants to have settled with us before He goes or they go. But God, just take it in your hands, and live with them. So, just do the best that you can Lord. Don't try to give them any kind of side warning or anything else, just give them a good clean bath so they can come to you in the heat of a good meal, and a good knowing, and a good reasoning to be there to pray with you Lord, and to hide under your duress Lord so that we can have the health and the bath that we need, Oh God. So, just be with us Lord and just keep Your hands over us. And let us be with You in all of this day. That we can feel your presence and your Holy Spirit and just bring it to us.

What this prayer reveals are the character and substance of her prayer life. Though she had come to the end of her Alzheimer's journey, her prayers remained theologically sound, biblically centered, and recipient-focused. The point is, in circumstances beyond our control, outside factors can take away our acquired knowledge and even the styles by which we demonstrate that knowledge, but they cannot take away our eternal relationship with the Lord. The Spirit always finds a way to speak to God on behalf of His people. The Apostle Paul described the miraculous nature of what we witnessed in these prayers in Romans 8:26-27 (NIV):

In the same way, the Spirit helps us in our weakness (Jeanette's cognitive impairment). We do not know what we ought to pray for (there was no way for her to understand), but the Spirit himself interceded for us with groans that words cannot express (the entry way to revelation, beyond the limitations of Alzheimer's disease). And he who searches our hearts knows the mind of the Spirit (even when her mental state and physical body were weak, her spirit remained willing), because the Spirit intercedes for the saints in accordance with God's will (the real and tangible expression of faith through prayer). [Commentary added.]

The best understanding I can give for what we witnessed in that latent stage of Alzheimer's is that Jeanette had chosen to abide in the presence of the Almighty and maintained a life fully submitted to the Spirit of God. That submitted spirit remained as the Lord continued to use her as an intercessor even when that was not medically probable. How? Love never fails. Jeanette loved the Lord, her God *and* her Neighbor, as herself.

This truth was present not only in her prayers but also in those times the family would gather for singing and worship. Toward the end of this final phase, when Jeanette had become immobile, we would gather around the bed or her wheelchair to sing some of her beloved hymns. In the midst of singing, she would raise her hands in worship and adoration, giving the Lord the honor and the glory He deserves. One of us would start the hymn and, as we finished the first stanza, a mostly static, (e)motionless Jeanette would join in singing vigorously. Often, she would take over singing the second and sometimes the third and fourth stanzas. It was as if the veil of disease was thrown back, momentarily, to allow the captive Jeanette to emerge as she worshipped the Lord her God. Some physicians would like to maintain the belief that by the final stage the old Jeanette would be completely gone. But I know—and my family bore witness—that the essence of who

193

Jeanette was remained. It had to; it was formed by the eternal hands of a Creator God. Alzheimer's can do its damage, but God through the Holy Spirit, maintains the integrity of the individual. She couldn't depart from her "self" because her identity wasn't built on the finite; it was formed out of the infinite. So what remained was that which remained—abided—in the Eternal Him.

Paradise Found

As I started this final stage, I felt like our paradise was being ripped from me. But from the rubble of her final stage she gave me a gift—a paradise found. It wasn't a paradise where we could take up residence; rather, it was an oasis she allowed us to visit occasionally with her, her childhood. In this final stage, Jeanette demonstrated on several occasions what I would call "the restoration of the joy of the child within her." As Jeanette experienced the Lord's sacrament of cleansing[46] and was released of all the social mores and pretenses of a very public life, she could finally express many deep, suppressed feelings not allowed by the *old Jeanette*. This

---

46 Of course, this "Sacrament of Cleansing" does not just apply to those with diseases in the general category of "dementia." Any major crisis, especially for the Christian, gives one the opportunity to take a serious look at all those experiences and achievements which we tenaciously cling to in order to decide which of these agendas are now relevant in light of this new covenant. While it may be initially difficult to praise the Lord for any crisis, we know from our histories, had it not been for a particular crisis, many of the good things the Lord had planned for us would have never happened. We Pentecostals have always known these facts existed. They existed, because, regardless of what happens to us in our crises of life, we always found a reason to rejoice. As my dear friend Dr. Steven J. Land says, "it is Pentecostal to cry and laugh at the same time."

unexpected and priceless gift was not just a gift for us (her family); it was a gift for Jeanette. Her crisis became her cleansing and her freedom. Not the old notion of *freedom from*, as many see spiritual freedom, but *freedom to*.[47] Freedom to pursue Him, unhindered. Freedom to love others without an agenda to tarnish it. And freedom to be uniquely us as created and inspired by the Creative Spirit of God. For Jeanette experienced in her cleansing, a freedom to experience without apology a childlikeness she was not afforded in her home of ten children. By her own account, she was forced into adulthood all too quickly, leaving her to feel as though she had been robbed of her childhood. Being the middle of ten kids, she was the primary one to make the sacrifices for the family. She was even taken out of school for one full year just to assist with this heavy burden. So when she moved into this final stage, she was granted the opportunity to restore some of what was lost in those early years. On many occasions, this playful Jeanette would replace the more serious and controlled Jeanette that we all knew.

> *Her crisis became her cleansing and her freedom.*

About a year prior to her death, the grandkids found her old high school baton. Jeanette loved to tell the story of the time her very restrictive parents allowed her to be a majorette with the high school band for one year. Unfortunately, after that season was up, she was

---

47 Karl Barth, "The Gift of Freedom: Foundations of Evangelical Ethics," in The Humanity of God. (Louisville: Westminster John Knox Press, translation, 1996), https://archive.org/details/TheHumanityOfGod-KarlBarth.

forced to return to her many household duties and, to her dissatisfaction, would never again be allowed to be a part of any other extra-curricular activities. Her work at home took precedence over everything else. Revisiting this uncommon season of youthful joy was a treat for all of us. The grandkids were especially overjoyed by this newly discovered image of their Oma as a young and playful majorette—an image that didn't line up with the sick and aging Oma who sat before them. Then, suddenly, something stirred in her, and for a few wonderful moments she grabbed the baton and gracefully gave us a flawless performance we would never forget. I can still see her twisting and turning, rotating the baton with precision between her fingers, throwing it in the air and gracefully catching it without missing a step. She pranced around the living room not like a woman in her eighties, but with the skill and beauty of a seventeen-year-old giving the performance of her life during the high school half-time celebration with the band. It was as if the limitations of age were temporarily lifted and she was given the freedom to live in the eternal now—outside of age and time.

> *Suddenly something stirred in her, and for a few wonderful moments she grabbed the baton and gracefully gave us a flawless performance we would never forget.*

Mesmerized by her play, we were all transformed into a fixed time where Jeanette experienced a great freedom and joy in her life which would certainly be short-lived and most certainly a loss she would not have been given permission (nor the time) to grieve. But that day, the Lord restored unto her the joy of a childhood lost. On that day and many others, the playful, "free to" Jeanette replaced the more serious Jeanette; more like our grandchildren whose child-like behavior surprised all of us on many occasions. In fact, that day marked the beginning of a paradise already found and not yet fully experienced for her.

This new found freedom to be young and joyful, outside of the cares of aging adulthood, provided us with so many other wonderful experiences with her too. As a young person (in her mind), her relationship with me greatly transformed. Our relationship was more akin to that of a grandfather and granddaughter. In her dependency, she let me be her entertainer, her considerably older friend and much needed presence. I would often spend hours making up and singing little lyrics to her. In those silly songs I would recount experiences from her earliest years with her mom and dad. She would smile real big, reach over and touch my arm, hold my hands, and clap like a little girl watching some entertaining event.

Breakfast also became a very special time with her. This was our time. For me it was the opportunity to revisit our early years when I was trying to romance her. Her very protective dad was suspicious of me, not allowing us to even hold hands in his presence. Though, at times, we violated his oversight. This was my last chance and long overdue time of continuing to romance the one I had loved all these years. Sometimes this special breakfast scene would go on for a couple hours. It was our fun, "give-and-take" time. Once I asked her if she would have ever considered dating someone like me. Her answer was quick and witty with a big, flirty smile, "Lord, no! If I did, my dad would kill me!"

The Lord was teaching me how to communicate with this previously suppressed "child within" her. I learned how to speak her language through my many made up lyrics which I would sing to her, like: "I met a girl on the side of the road, painting her bright red toes" or "You are more beautiful than a rose; and if I had my choice, you would be the sweetheart of my soul." Her big responses always encouraged my efforts. Once, she even leaned over and kissed the back of my hand. Gaining a degree of trust and approval, I felt in those moments, in a small measure, I had entered into her Alzheimer's land and was speaking her Alzheimer's language. Little did I know this entry into her child-like state was only weeks from the conclusion of her long struggle with Alzheimer's.

In the Lord's plan for all of us, while He takes, He also restores. Nothing illustrates this better than that passage in Mark 10: 15-16: "I tell you the truth, anyone who will not receive the Kingdom of God like a little child will never enter it. And, He took the children in His arms, put His hands on them and blessed them." None of us rejoiced with the loss of the "old Jeanette," the perfected manager of all our lives who carefully and attentively watched over us with a dutiful sense of personal responsibility. But neither did we reject this new, more child-like Jeanette. It was the Lord's way of teaching us to celebrate the entire story of our lives—that which was, what is, and that which is to be found.

Finally, toward the end of her physical battle with Alzheimer's, Jeanette experienced what her neurologist determined to be undetected mini-strokes, resulting in her having to be more carefully monitored around the clock. Then, approximately three months before she died, she fell. From that point on, she lost the use of her limbs. It was clear the end was very near. Though it may seem strange, we waited fearfully and reverently with an expectation that something wonderful was about to happen.

Making Sense of Jeanette's Final Phase

The significance of Jeanette's journey for my life begins with the sacramental cleansing that took place along the way. I had been a Christian, a minister, a chaplain, professor, clinical supervisor, and so much more; yet God, in his infinite wisdom, saw fit to clean up this old chaplain from the burdens and the defilement of ministering in a broken world. It was my duty to reach and touch the untouchable, and it was my privilege to let God reach and touch me. His cleansing qualified me (and Jeanette) to shift from one spiritual condition to the next; it is what allowed me to remain with her as long as I did and to maintain covenantal integrity rather than digress to a more contractual relationship. *(In saying this, I mean no condemnation to the many families who—for many reasons—are unable to join their companion or parent in a similar manner. I recognize the great privilege I was given to be released from all other heavy responsibilities to give almost total attention to this one single task. I did it because I felt it was both for Jeanette's best interest and for mine. And, I saw this as the last opportunity for me to journey with her as a full participant in her battle with Alzheimer's.)* Of course, for me this "covenant" would require her to be cared for at home and in close care partnership with our family, our local church, and the countless others who assisted me.

My decision came very early in the process. When I made this firm commitment, little did I know that the process would give us new identities appropriate for her last journey from earth to paradise; nor did I know the process would require my own transformative cleansing in order to remain joined to her on the journey. Once relieved of all those previous attachments and identities, the Lord showed me something I could not have anticipated this late in my life: preparation for a new ministry. It was as if he had granted me, like Sarai and Elizabeth, the ability to produce beyond my expected age. Don't get me wrong, I wasn't waiting for an unfulfilled promise. God had granted me a life greater than I could have conceived for myself. Yet He wasn't finished with me. Like Sarai and Elizabeth, my age didn't disqualify me; submission to His stripping, cleansing, and a new and uncomfortable path qualified me. And it is what continues to qualify me.

In many ways my process paralleled Jacob's (Genesis 32: 22-32), who found himself wrestling with the Lord throughout the night, holding on for dear life demanding the Lord bless him. Instead, the Lord gave this future leader a new identity. He no longer would be known as Jacob, but Israel, because he struggled with God and men and won. Others may call this an optimal time of decision-making: a *Kairos* moment. These are the times when the winds shift, and we find ourselves at a critical decision-making moment so important that our life, depending on which decision we make, will never be the same. From my perspective as a Christian, I had already made my choice. Jeanette and I had taken many journeys together in our sixty plus years of marriage, family and ministries. No matter what the call, Jeanette joined me at each of those ministry and family junctures with her own unique identity and assignments.

In the end, when she was so helpless, I was privileged to be the caregiver she wanted and depended upon. As she got closer to the end, only a select few were granted access to the door of her new land and language as she transitioned from the *land of Alzheimer's* to Paradise. I cherished this role and, for that matter, all the roles she gave to me. At first I misunderstood my role; I needed to fix her. As I better understood the disease and its progression, I realized my role was to be whatever she needed me to be in every given moment. I also discovered that my own disposition had a lot to do with what she saw my role to be. If I was upset, then naturally she would name me as someone unpleasant—a lesson I tried to pass on to all those who cared for her. Jeanette, even in this advanced stage, could quickly tell if I or someone else approached their responsibilities as a "duty" rather than an "act of love" for her. I do not know how she could distinguish that, but she did. Caregivers and visitors who came to visit or care for her were instructed on: how to talk to her, give eye contact with her, listen to her, not get in a hurry to respond, and not to reject any feelings she gave to them. Most importantly, they were to receive her perception as reality, at least for that given moment of personal contact. Accepting her perception is the price one pays to get beyond the front door of her heart and into her world and her language, where she lives at that moment in time.

Of course, this is not her permanent home. Give it a little time and you will realize, too, that this earthly life is just your journey inspired by a Divine Mission. It is a part of God's cleansing ritual which takes us from this earthly world to paradise, His eternal residence.

Chaplains, Friends and Ministerial Colleagues:

I am sending this letter to you with very mixed emotions. First, I know that most of you are at the General Assembly. How I wish I could have joined you and once again hugged the necks of our hundreds of chaplains, their spouses, and their kids. As you know, I will always have those "daddy and granddaddy" feelings in regards to this wonderful chaplaincy family. I do hope to see you soon at other special events. And, who knows, I may unexpectedly show up at your military base, prison, hospital, CSC sites, and all those other places where the Church of God's best give their sacrificial love and care to those in need.

Now, let me share my deepest and abiding emotion: my love and devotion to a wonderful wife, mother, and grand-mother: none other than Katherine Jeanette Crick. Jeanette is now officially a client with Hospice. She is still at home, but receiving 24-hour care. Just today, she went into a deep coma-like state. She has very little to eat or drink and is on a "Hospice watch" for the next couple days. Basically, Hospice, with my participation, has decided to let her and the Lord lead; and we will follow, accepting the outcome as from our loving Lord. If she does come out of this present crisis, we will continue to do what we do around the clock: love her, joke with her, recount with her all those big and little events of our 65 years of marriage and more than 57 years of ministry. She loves to have me read the Scriptures, sing the old "red back" hymns, pray with her until the Holy Spirit fills the room with His presence, and (though seldom able to complete her thoughts with understandable words) lift those boney arms upward in the middle of my prayers and speak prayerfully in that wonderful heavenly language. Are we not all thrilled that this language of the Spirit remains with us right as we leave this world and step into that heavenly world?

I promise you that if and when the Lord takes her, you will be notified immediately. I boldly state that when the Lord lets this happen, I will need every one of you: your prayers, embrace, and, if possible, your presence. I cannot imagine any of us making our journey from earth to heaven without the presence and support of our chaplaincy family.

Finally, please continue to pray for us, especially as Jeanette goes through what Hospice defines as her final stages. We do not see it that way; it is not "final" with us. It is simply just another step with the Lord, having nearly finished one phase of His Journey and getting ready, with a deep abiding peace and joy, for another phase. Remember, it is not accidental that you are receiving this newsletter. Your faces are burned into our hearts as a reminder we are "never alone." I would not want it any other way. Blessings to your families and all those who depend on your ministry. Only eternity will tell how our chaplaincy family has impacted our church and our world. Thanks for accepting such a lofty "call and ministry." God Bless.

Newsletter, Bob and Jeanette Crick, 7/31/2014[48]

---

48   This is one of many newsletters sent out to families, friends, and colleagues during the course of her sickness. It was the easiest and most efficient way to update everyone on Jeanette's progress. It was also how I stayed connected to those people we loved and depended on for moral and spiritual support. These correspondences made our journey seem less isolated from the world we could less and less be a part of.

Chapter 9

Freedom in Forgiveness: Releasing My Treasure to be Stored in Heaven

"Healthy children will not fear life
If their elders have integrity enough not to fear death."
—*Erik H. Erikson*[49]

The end of Jeanette's journey into the land and language of Alzheimer's came all too quickly. I know now that a part of me was in a state of denial, crying within, "Lord, don't let it end!" By then my covenant to be with her in this journey was so strong that I think my preference would have been to hold on to her until it was my time to take my final journey as well. I know this isn't logical, nor something Jeanette would have wanted. We had that typical, pragmatic understanding about this last phase of our life. Whoever lived on must live life to the uttermost as a testimony of God's grace and sustaining power. But that all goes away as you

---

49   Quote By Erik H. Erikson. Quotery. n.d. Sat. 5 Dec. 2015. <http://www.quotery.com/quotes/healthy-children-will-not-fear-life-if-their-elders-have/>.

watch the love of your life deteriorate, fragment by fragment. Logic is not logical in those moments of intense grief. I could not bear to think of her leaving me so soon. And I certainly could not bear the thought of continuing what had always been *our journey* without her, even in her weakened state.

The deterioration was obvious. Her body was frail. Over a period of less than a year her weight went from about 120 pounds down to less than 100. To deal with my feelings, I would joke with her saying, "Whoa, Jeanette, my beauty, you are now at the weight when we first met and I married you in 1948." In those days she weighed a meager 105 pounds, and I loved every pound of her. So I did what any man impaired by love would do: I pleaded with the Lord to let me hold on to her just a little bit longer.

> *My heart told me that this was going to be the most excruciating reality I would ever endure.*

My heart told me that this was going to be the most excruciating reality I would ever endure. For all these years, through all our sundry experiences, Jeanette was always there for me in a powerful and sustaining way. I trusted her faithfulness not only to me, but especially to the Lord. She was the first person I called on for prayer when I faced a new responsibility or change in station. We were a team, and a good team depends on the unique gifts that each member brings with them—even their differences. Jeanette and I both had strong personalities; we had differences and were very comfortable expressing those differences. However, we had lived together long enough to know when to call on the unique gifting which one or the other possessed in abundance. This is how effective teams operate; to us, that was just smart business. Why struggle when right at your disposal you could say, without any misunderstanding, "Honey, this is more in your territory. Help me out." What terrified me at the core was how incomplete I would be without my most significant teammate. Though I knew she had already "left the team," in my heart she was still very present in spite of her fragmented physical state. My heart was out of control; I was desperate, despairing—even resistant to the realities of her impending death. I was fully convinced I could not be whole without my cherished covenant partner. I had invested so much in our covenant; how do I exist in its absence? Who will I be once it is broken? Helpless in my emotional wanderings, I exhausted myself wondering if it would ever be restored again. I had so much more to learn about God's covenant, and the Lord was patient in my slow learning. Eventually, though, it would begin to sink in as well for me... .

May 25th, 2014: The Beginning of Goodbye

Some of the answers to these lingering, powerful questions came during one of our final, private sharing times together. It was a Sunday evening, three months before she left us for Paradise. I do not know how, but she was able to talk and pray with more clarity than I had experienced with her in several weeks. It was as if, just for this special occasion, she was somewhat her old self. The moment with her was timeless; the conversation was sobering. We shared freely and unrepentantly our fears and our unconditional love for one another. My heart was wide open. In my transparency and vulnerability, she responded with a seemingly unusual understanding. I told her with hardly any hesitation or restrictions my fears of losing her. I cried openly and unashamedly; several times she reached over to comfort me in my grief. Uncertain at times if she really knew who I was, I readily accepted her gift of love and compassion. Maybe I needed it more than I needed to be known.

In the conversation I asked her if she had any fears of dying and leaving us. As if she hadn't a concern in this world, she pleasantly replied, "No. Whatever the Lord wants, I want." I told her of my fears; again, she showed not one bit of fear, only pure, holy resignation. I told her how much I would miss her, and she smiled as if to say, "That's nice. Thank you." I am so glad I opened myself to her in that way, for I had held in my emotions for so long. I needed to tell her those sacred and fearful feelings while she was with me. These were feelings I had kept private since the moment we received her terminal diagnosis. I had wanted to be so positive, working through all the phases with such optimism. I was the cheerleader for the family, our caregivers, and even for the medical staff. But, this was my time to be absolutely human, and I knew I could not be that vulnerable with any other person other than my devoted Jeanette.

As the conversation transitioned into our devotion time, a third presence joined our private moment. I know it was the work of the Holy Spirit when I chose Matthew chapter six. I read the whole chapter about caring for those in need, prayer, and fasting. When I reached verses 19-21, I knew why we were sharing this scripture together. It came so naturally. There, as if chosen just for me, were the words:

> *Do not store up for yourself treasures on earth, where moth and rust destroy and where thieves break in and steal. But store up for yourselves treasures in heaven, where moth and rust do not destroy, and where thieves do not break in and steal. For where your treasure is, there your heart will be also. (NIV)*

The voice of the Spirit could not have been clearer. Jeanette was my treasure, and the Lord was telling me to release this treasure to be stored in heaven. Being so poor growing up, struggling just for the light of day, I always clung tightly to everything I received. In my heart, I pled with God: *I know you are the God who gives and takes away. But, I found her. I worked hard to earn her heart, and I will never give her up! I can't give her up; she is my life's treasure. Please, don't be the God who takes away!* The Lord was trying to teach me something very powerful, not only for this moment, but for the days ahead. However, I couldn't receive because I could not let go yet. It wasn't until after Jeanette had died that I realized how carefully the Lord was orchestrating, for both of us, this final departure. He was telling me that these earthly experiences, cleansed by the Word and the Holy Spirit, were not treasures to hold onto. By releasing them, they would be stored in the only place where they— she—would live eternally.

Finally, I asked Jeanette if she would pray for me. I just felt this may be my last chance for her final blessings. She readily agreed. I am so thankful I recorded that prayer. Let me share verbatim, so that you can feel both the advanced effects of the disease on her words and, most importantly, the depth of her words as she blessed me:

> *Father, tonight we come to You because we know You are the One that takes God at His best and will give to us His wisdom to go into the place of the people—to give them the things that God alone can give to them.*
>
> *And Father help him (me) to understand tonight; give to him the Holy Spirit so he will know when to do and what to say. O God, that he would live so before the Lord so that they (the people) will all know what this man has been able to do.*
>
> *God, we just ask that he (me) would take your best system, and that this servant of the Lord would stand before You, and give him the life and wisdom so for us to stand before them (the people).*
>
> *Father, just touch him and give him the wisdom that he will need to do and use to stand face-to-face before God and the people. Just reach forth and let the people be taught the ways of Your wisdom. Help them to come before You and give themselves to You, O Lord; give them the grace to take care of Your wisdom because your family is in the wisdom of God.*

Father, keep Your wisdom, life and joy for the people living with You. And touch him and guide him, letting him taste Your wisdom, life and ways. Let us taste of the wisdom of these babies that the Lord has produced. O God, reach down and touch this man when he comes before You, Lord, so when he comes into this place to become one of the ones You have taught.

When she finished, I declared with a strong affirmation, "Amen!" She followed with an equally strong, "Amen, Papa!"

May 29: Closures with Honors

Jeanette and I were honored and blessed in many ways during our last three months together. On May 29, we were inducted into the Seminary's Hall of Prophets. Induction into the Hall of Prophets is reserved for ministers whose service to Jesus Christ and the Church has been meritorious. A very important feature of the Hall of Prophets is the establishment of a scholarship in honor of the nominee which will be a constant source of funding for students preparing for ministry. Hundreds of people shared in this special day. I spoke of the many years of raising a good family, grand-kids who loved their Oma, and all the various assignments and achievements we shared together. Students, professors, chaplains, and friends blessed us with testimonies of how personal their relationships had been with us. They noted time and again Jeanette's personal, private ways of blessing them behind the scenes through

211

funds, prayers, and loving counsel. And how she did so without any fanfare.

All three of our kids gave their own prepared videos with very personal, warm remarks of how Jeanette had guided them during their lifetime. She was the "mother hen" whose love was never doubted. Though a marvelous event, it was bittersweet. Jeanette was unable to make the 130-mile trip. There I was trying to hold back tears, in an event that should never be experienced alone. This was our day. We ministered faithfully together. I wanted her to see how God had given us His affirming nod, validating the sacrificial life that comes with the vocation of ministry. I wanted them to see her, see her role, validate her part in that long story of service. So I made her present by telling her story and our story whenever possible.

When I described to Jeanette all the hundreds who came to the ceremony, followed by a great meal and hours of fellowship, with testimony after testimony of her personal love and care for so many, she simply responded, "That's nice. That's nice."

Through the eyes of her daughter Jonne:

Life without Mom's direction proved more challenging than I had realized. Our dependence on her was always more notable in these times. In many ways, she was the director of our family in both small and large ways. Dad called me to his hotel room the morning of the induction. With three ties in hand, he said, "Your Mom always picked out what I should wear, but she's not here to do it for me. Can you tell me which tie looks best?" My heart was saddened. This was Mom's job, not mine. I picked out a tie I thought that Mom would have approved. Dad then asked me to help set up the display table outside the chapel once we arrived at the seminary, which I was delighted to do. As I sifted through all the pictures of Mom and Dad in various ministries and all the boxes of awards and plaques of recognition, I struggled and became overwhelmed trying to set it up. This is something Mom would have normally done with ease, and done it perfectly. But for me, it was a struggle to make it just right. Thankfully, some of the staff at the seminary saw my struggles and stepped in to help. The display was not as perfect as it would have been had Mom done it, but we did our best to honor her!

First Week of June: Healing for the Wounded

The first week of June, I made a short trip to Romania for a very special book signing and conference with hundreds of pastors and family members. The book was a Romanian contextual translation of my book, *Outside the Gates.* A highlight of the conference came with me sharing Jeanette's Alzheimer's journey. I told them about the many phases of Alzheimer's, the ups and downs of that journey, and the emotional fatigue that accompanies this kind of enduring illness. Most importantly, I explained how we eventually submitted our envisioned ending to the Lord's perfectly scripted ending. In doing so, I assured them this was no easy task. But our trust is inevitably in the Lord.

This theme hit a common chord among the participants, bringing a measure of closure not only for me in my suffering, but for the countless others whose lives have been touched by so much pain and loss. Many of these older Romanian pastors had suffered greatly during the Soviet Union's forty-four year occupation of Romania. They understood suffering and readily identified with Jeanette's long battle with this terrible disease and impending death. They also identified with me, her lifelong family and ministry partner, as I told them the pain of anticipating giving her up. Additionally, I was able to share with them this precious Jeanette.

By conference call, I piped in recordings of her praying for us prior to leaving the US with Jonne's help. While her thoughts seem too disjointed to recover any significant meaning, when you see much deeper than the surface, a profound message emerges from the rubble. Her prayer is a prayer of empowerment. From the beginning, she calls on God to draw us carefully into His safety nest only to push us forward into flight. He equips and makes us righteous. By drawing us in, transforming us, and touching our hands, He sends us out to be used by Him for His glory and to accomplish His great mission in us. To which, she rightly responds, *we praise you and we do glorify you, Lord!*

April 9, 2014

Father, we know that You are the One that is the One that has taken care of us, and taken, Oh God, into the nest of all that is here. And Father, You are the One who has done all things that has been pushed forward tonight. And we know you are the One that has taken our lives, so we praise you so much for that. And Father, we know the joy that you've given to us for over all of this, Father. Father, just take your hands and move over them, and let him know that You were the One that was the One that moved into his life, and gave his help to You. And God we also know that You were the One who helped him (speaking of me in Romania) to bring the life of the people that You have turned into rightness. And God we do glorify You and thank you so much over all of that, Lord. But Lord we do ask that You would touch our hands, and that you would use us Lord, to do for You, what You have already done for people today.

She goes on for another five minutes before ending the prayer with a singular focus: our need for more of God to be present in and near us. This closing was lifted up specifically for the Romanian people who attended the conference and for me:

Father, just let him (me) to know your love and your mercy. And Oh, God just hold Yourself before him and let him feel You, Lord. That thing is joy that he would like to have tonight. So Lord just reach over to him and touch him. We trust you Lord, and we trust the life that You have already given to him. And Father just touch him, and just give him love and mercy. And help him to keep his life cemented to you, Lord. Just move with him and help him, Oh God, to voice his love to you. In Jesus's Holy name we ask it all, in the name of Jesus Christ, in our lives. We do enjoy you, Father, for what you do for us, and what You give us, and what you can tell us, and what you can help us to understand. Lord we do ask you to be with us through this day, and through this anointing in Jesus's Holy Name. Amen.

Her prayers touched a common chord and led all of us into a time of prayer. God was so near to us in our brokenness. We "knew" this to be true, but that moment of in-breaking was so powerful it moved us to that wonderful, profound experience of Awe. That place where knowledge becomes realized through the experience of revelation. Then the Lord began to break in on the hushed silence of our hearts. That "hush" that causes us to plead *not now, not here;* that hush which keeps us locked up and never *free to.* The conference leader, sensing the move of the Spirit, stepped in and began to lead all of us into a time of prayer for those suffering with this or other illnesses and their love ones. As we prayed together, the presence of the Almighty permeated the auditorium with healing, comfort, encouragement, and renewed strength. It became a time of breaking the silence as we loved one another and shared with each other. Several times the Holy Spirit manifested himself powerfully, with voices and utterances more precious than life itself. I could not have anticipated that this simple conference would bring such a blessed time of healing, renewal, and closure for my own journey with Jeanette. Praise be to the Sovereign God, Most High!

The only answer I could give as to *why this conference* is to borrow from author Henri Nouwen. In Nouwen's book, *The Wounded Healer*, he concludes:

> ...*it has become clear that Christian leadership is accomplished only through service. This service requires the willingness to enter into a situation, with all the human vulnerabilities a man has to share with his fellow man. This is a painful and self-denying experience, but an experience which can indeed lead man out of his prison of confusion and fear. Indeed, the paradox of Christian leadership is that the way out is the way in that only by entering into communion with human suffering can relief be found.*[50]

Without any real intention on my part to do so, I entered into the pain of others by way of my own pain and story. The brokenness of my spirit, which only began a couple weeks earlier as I confessed my fears and anguish to Jeanette, became my door of hope in a valley of great crisis. As I acknowledged how ravished my heart was by the anticipated loss of Jeanette, we were all granted permission to grieve, weep, be honest about where we were in our own healing processes, reach out to one another, and reach up to receive an authentic touch from God. That afternoon, as we opened ourselves before God and others, we became Christ with flesh... incarnate, wounded healers. Thus, we were transformed by His revelatory

---

50 Henri Nouwen, The Wounded Healer: Ministry in Contemporary Society (New York: Doubleday Dell Publishing Group, Inc., 1972), 77.

presence and, consequently, entered into the healing process. This happened because in that moment we decided to not shy away from our pain, but acknowledge it, give it words and witnesses. In so doing, those words made available the grace and mercy of God to both the giver (maybe, in this case, *the gifter*) and the recipient of care.

June 19: The End is Near

On June 19, 2014, my family met with Hospice personnel to set up a care plan for Jeanette's last days. This final care experience was all too short. Even with the best of care, the end was imminent. We could sense it, and Jeanette could also sense it. For the most part she seemed to simply run out of reasons to remain with us. She was so resigned to the path she was on, it seemed her message to us was: *You have done all you need to do, let me go.* I knew she was tired of that old body. It had become a weight too great for her to carry. I sensed that she longed for that promised *new body* and to be clothed in His glory rather than the worn out earthly vessel which besieged her. This final process was like a woman giving birth. The "birthing pains" which would ultimately lead to her deliverance from that earthly shell, came more quickly and remained longer. While she was waiting with eager expectation (Rom. 8: 18-21) to be liberated from her present state and delivered into the arms of her Abba Father, we simply waited, silently groaning in our confusion and suffering.

July 9: Broken by a Fall

Another birthing pain came on July 9. She fell, possibly due to a stroke. Dale rushed to her side. Yet in her newfound resolve, as any mother in the throes of deliverance, her concern was for him. She tried to comfort him, saying, "Dale, son, I am okay. Please, son, I am okay." Because our finite minds could not yet comprehend nor detect the grand metamorphosis taking place before us, her seemingly disjointed response was actually the most precise. The most obvious interpretation of the moment was that she was okay; we were the ones broken by the fall.

In these final weeks, Jeanette was surrounded by those who mattered the most to her: her kids and grandkids. When one of them entered into the room, she would give them a tired but meaningful smile. Most fortunately, Jonne arrived a day after Jeanette's fall and injury. She had, again, taken time off from work to care for her mom around the clock and for me as I recovered from hernia surgery. When we would offer her our gratitude, she would simply say, "I am so honored to return to both of you the love and care of the nature which you have given me over the years." From her own reflections, Jonne later shared with me these words:

> *Because our finite minds could not yet comprehend nor detect the grand metamorphosis taking place before us, her seemingly disjointed response was actually the most precise. She was okay; we were the ones broken by the fall.*

I am so fortunate to have gotten Mom's sweet and loving responses in her final days. During these precious experiences, Mom would lay her head on my shoulder and her hands on my chest. She would allow me to massage her feet and legs. It was a gift I willingly received as I felt the healing and acceptance between us…

As the situation progressed toward its natural conclusion, her body could no longer perform consistently its many necessary duties. Her internal organs were closing down. We were dealing more and more with kidney infections, constipation, diarrhea, stomach disorders, and other illnesses related to this disease. She ran a low grade fever and had lost her desire or need for food. All of us, family and caregivers, were determined that she would get a proper, nutritious diet. When she lost the ability to chew, we pureed her foods, knowing that she would refuse most of what we offered her. Nevertheless, in our desire to keep her with us, we denied these signs believing them to be only temporary. So we maintained our focus on the original goal: giving Jeanette the finest, most loving care possible.

August: The End is Here

A couple weeks before she died, thinking this is the "hour," the family surrounded her bed. Rachel, our granddaughter, jumped on the bed and sang Oma's favorite song, "Over the Rainbow." Jonah, our grandson, hugged her, prayed with her, and told her, through his many tears, how much she meant to him. Rachel, overcome by the significance of the moment, began crying uncontrollably for her Oma. Trying to calm her down, Jonah repeatedly stated, "Look, Rachel. She is not dead, yet. She is moving her toes!"

All of us felt this would be her last hour, but it wasn't. For a few more days we were able to sporadically communicate with her. It was as if the Lord brought her back to us so that we could appropriately thank her for those many years of faithful service and ministry as Mom, Oma, Sister, Friend, and, of course my Blessed Wife. Knowing in my heart that we were at the end, I would send our caregivers to bed so I could lie next to her throughout the night. Together in our bed, I would hold her hand, pray with her, and sing softly to my "little sweetheart" as she would slip in and out of a deep-sleep pattern. She received it graciously, often holding tightly to my hand or arm as she went into a deep sleep. Of course, by now Hospice was encouraging us to give her more morphine sulfate to ease her pain. They also advised us not to give her food or water. This was most painful for all the family. We felt like we were starving to death the one we loved the most.

That last week or so was not without some tension, especially with me. I became increasingly irritable dealing with all the many facets of managing her end of life care as well as my own experience of grief. I was tired, angry, lonely for my wife, and so sad. My grief and anger were close to the surface as I anticipated saying goodbye to the love of my life. And I was certainly less tolerant of outsiders with uninformed opinions about her care. For instance, one of Jeanette's relatives came for a visit. Unfortunately, I wasn't home at the time. While visiting, she got involved in a conflict with one of our primary caregivers. She so upset the care process that the caregiver wanted to leave immediately. Once informed of the incident, I got the relative on the phone and asked her to depart. I realized at that point how much my grief and anger had grown. As was often the case, persons visiting did not understand what it was like to care for someone with this disease, and not just for days, but years.

Many of these "visitors" would give their quick opinions in regards to how we were caring for Jeanette and, in a few cases, questioned our lack of faith for healing. For this reason, primary caregivers must use Godly wisdom in dealing with these "outsiders." Jesus said it best on the cross, "Forgive them, Father, for they know not what they do." Those "non-caregiver" family and friends do not understand the kind of care necessary for loved ones like Jeanette. In their ignorance, they believe they have a better solution to the disease or care plan and offer unhelpful insight. So, though a great cross to bear, the caregivers must not only extend their energies toward the care recipient, but to those peripheral participants who lack understanding. A way to prevent some of that tension is to be proactive in these visits. First, the primary caregiver must be patient with these visitors, not expecting them to have a deep understanding of the disease and its many physical, social, and spiritual dimensions. Second, the caregiver should take time, even before the visit, to lovingly and gently give instructions to the visitor(s) as to the best way to communicate, pray, and interact with their loved one—especially those with Alzheimer's disease. In this manner, the caregiver is both protecting the visitor and the loved one.[51] Finally, patience and forgiveness must also be reserved for all of us caregivers, too. Anger is an appropriate first reaction for the overburdened caregiver. Spiritually, it is just that, a first reaction. The follow up to anger is understanding, love, and eventually partnership (when possible) with family members, caregivers, medical professionals and visitors. We needed everyone to assist and to keep the focus on the main issue: the best care possible for Jeanette in her final days with us.

Of course, Jeanette would not be Jeanette if she didn't participate in the caregiving in some way. With so little left to offer, she gave all that remained to her beloved children, and they willingly and openly received her love. David wept for nearly 30 minutes with his head on her chest. Her final gift of love was to comfort him and embrace him one last time with her hands on his head. It was truly a mother/son moment. Dale was constantly at her bedside holding her hand, with a deep look of love and concern, holding back his tears. And Jonne lay beside her, talking with her, and letting her know how much she loved her mom (even in a nearly unconscious state).

Then there were the grandkids. Even in her barely conscious state, she always opened her eyes and smiled when the grandkids would enter. She seemed to have never forgotten their names and

---

51   It may also be beneficial for the visitor to know the scope of this disease. Eventually this and similar diseases will affect in some measure every household, worldwide. Aging, death and dying, and diseases in the general category of "dementia" are now a permanent fixture for all of us to face. Due to a number of factors, our general population is living longer, thus making all of us more aware that as we grow older we are more likely to be a candidate for Alzheimer's and other similar diseases.

special place in her life. They did not care what the protocol was; this was Oma, who understood them and accepted then just like they are. All five were present: Rachel and Jonah (nine-year-old twins); Samantha (five years old); and Dylan and Mackenzie (three-year-old twins). They came with so much energy and joy. In those final days, they shared with Oma their toys, songs, and drawings, but most of all, they shared their love. The expressions on Jeanette's face told what she was feeling in her final hours with her beloved grandkids. She was released from this long and complicated journey with Alzheimer's into a new Kingdom equated with the simplicity and depth of the virtues of childhood found in Matthew 18: 1-5 (NIV):

> *At that time the disciples came to Jesus and asked, "Who is the greatest in the kingdom of heaven?" He called a little child and had him stand among them. And he said: "I tell you the truth, unless you change and become like little children, you will never enter the kingdom of heaven. Therefore, whoever humbles himself like this child is the greatest in the kingdom of heaven. And whoever welcomes a little child like this is the greatest in the kingdom of heaven."*

August 22: Her Final Benediction

On Friday, August 22, three days before she died, Jeanette's family members from California visited her. To our surprise, she was able to talk to most of them, briefly and with broken sentences. She seemed to recognize them. After a short while, she asked clearly that Dale be sent to her. He came in the room, asked her if she was in any pain. She answered clearly, "No." As he continued talking, in the same way she had dealt with her kids over the years, she focused on his eyes, and said, "Son, you hush." She closed her eyes and like an old soldier who had fought long and hard, she readied herself for an eternal rest. Little did we know these words "you hush," would be her final, clearly understood words to all of us. Though only two words, in my heart I heard them as, *Be quiet, my beloved, the end is here, embrace it with Holy Silence.*

Following these final sacred moments with her immediate and extended family, Jeanette went into a deep, coma-like state. Jonne and I, along with Linda, one of our caregivers, were with her as her body began to shake and twist. Then without warning, she began to vomit violently. Her bowels exploded with unbelievable discharges, one after another. It was as if her body was emptying itself of all remaining impurities in preparation for that final journey from earth to Paradise.

Many came to visit us in those last days: her brothers and sisters, her nieces and nephews, friends, chaplains, peers, co-workers, and church family. Jeanette's departure is so characteristic of what is described in Hebrews 12: 1-3 (NIV):

> *Therefore, since we are surrounded by such a great cloud of witnesses, let us throw off everything that hinders and the sin that so easily entangles, and let us run with perseverance the race marked out for us. Let us fix our eyes on Jesus, the author and perfector of our faith, who by the joy set before him endured the cross, scorning its shame, and sat down at the right hand of the throne of God.*

That, as far as I am concerned, is her final Benediction. She had faithfully raised up a standard for her family and her ministry, thrown off everything that hindered her, fixed her eyes on Christ Jesus, and now she was ready to run that final race alone. With spiritual eyes, I envisioned angels running along each side of her. This was no longer a race *toward* Alzheimer's; rather it was a race *through* Alzheimer's and *to* the very arms of a loving Lord.

> *This was no longer a race toward Alzheimer's; rather it was a race through Alzheimer's and to the very arms of a loving Lord.*

During that weekend, from Friday evening until Monday morning, I dismissed all the caregivers leaving our precious Mom, Grandmother and Wife with the immediate family she so greatly treasured over the years. Due to the morphine, she was in and out of consciousness. Occasionally she would move or quietly groan. But most of the time she was in a deep, deep sleep.

August 25: Her Death

The last few hours of care included all of us doing all we could to make Jeanette's departure a deeply meaningful one. She never lacked for anything. Yet in her final state, she wanted nothing more than her immediate family in her presence. She died peacefully on Monday morning, August 25, 2014, at 3:30 a.m. with me lying by her side. When I realized she was gone, my heart broke. I hugged her and thanked her for 66 years of faithfulness, love, devotion, and passion for the Lord. I knew my soul and heart would never be the same. As I lingered in our last moments together, I realized that the greatest challenge the Lord would ever give me was to live on without my faithful partner. I was dazed by the all too surreal moment, a prolonged existential moment. It was as if this last instant found its way into our beloved reel-to-reels and was being played before me and not lived out in me. Not fully in the moment yet, I called for our kids.

I was in a trance that I couldn't break free from and I'm not sure I wanted to be freed. In a trance, it was someone else's reel-to-reel; it wasn't mine. Unable to enter into the moment, I just watched. I watched the Hospice nurse come to give the formal death time and cause; I remained silently stunned. I watched them take her beautiful body out of the room and load it onto the hearse, but I was silently, passively, stunned. This departure had temporally put my life, my emotions, and my soul on hold. I wanted to comfort the family, especially the kids and grandkids, but right then my soul was too empty to do anything.

That next day, the kids and I met to pick out the casket and make all the necessary funeral arrangements. Again I wanted to comfort them, but I could do nothing other than just the minimal administrative duties of preparing her obituary and arranging the funeral and graveside services. Fully stunned, my *reel all too real*, was nothing more than a foreign film without the luxury of subtitles. I heard them talking and agreed with the terms of the funeral and burial but my soul was still silent, impartial, and unable to grasp the magnitude of these final moments. Passively, I submitted to the rituals, but my heart could not put to rest that part of me too sacred to be touched by death. Accusingly, I asked: *Death, where is your sting?* I knew where it was. It was here. In the emptiness of my half person, my half soul. They say that only time will heal my pain. What happens when time refuses to advance itself? Stinging. Perpetual stinging.... .

August 28: The Funeral

The visitation and funeral were held at the North Cleveland Church of God on August 28, 2014. As we approached four o'clock, the parking lot filled with family after family. For two hours, hundreds waited patiently in line to pay their respects. Many long-term friends shared their love and deep admiration for my very "special lady." Their remembrances of her were true to her character, and I loved hearing them over and over. One after another gave the same testimony, "She was my blessing in times of crises."

> *Accusingly, I asked: Death, where is your sting? I knew where it was. It was here. In the emptiness of my half person, my half soul.*

In truth, she was a servant to so many and loved her role. She didn't do it to be seen, but always did it behind the scenes, keeping her left hand from knowing what the right hand had accomplished. Still, we saw...maybe not to this magnitude. But we all saw and felt the magnitude of her kindness toward each one of us. One military

228

chaplain testified: "I struggled in seminary. She would often assist me with my studies, with my finances, and even typing my dissertation at no cost. Without that help in my seminary education, I would never have been a career military chaplain." In truth, I had always known that she was a "great lady," but I had no idea the number of people she had ministered to formally and informally through the ministry of presence and care. She was a true servant of the Lord for both her family and the hundreds of people she faithfully served over the years.

Finally, we took our seats to begin the service. Several great speakers spoke on her behalf. I wish I could give an account of their words, but I couldn't hear over the static in my mind. The voices before me were indistinct and otherworldly. I still couldn't grasp them. I was both overwhelmed by an abundance of emotions and a void of emotions, too much and nothing all at the same time. It should have completely exhausted me, yet I felt like I should be doing something. Being still to listen seemed so out of place. I needed to help somebody, anybody, her...me. Tending to *her* bedside; telling *her* stories and singing *her* songs. I needed to make it all right. I needed to make it all right in me. Instead, I sat obediently and dutifully.

At the end of the hour-long service, Rachel sung her Oma's favorite song, "Over the Rainbow." Then all the kids joined me at the front of the altar for a time of personal sharing. As we closed the service, we honored her by singing "When We All Get to Heaven" from her most beloved song book, the old red-back hymnal. That was the last song I sang to her.

The graveside ceremony at the Chattanooga National Cemetery was, again, a stark reminder of both my life with Jeanette and my life without her. Some of our dearest friends gave final remarks of committal. I gave all present the opportunity to say a few words about their relationship with Jeanette. Several spoke, but it was Jonah, our grandson, who captured the significance of this sacred moment. Standing at the head of her casket waving his arms to get our attention, he stated with all the conviction a nine-year-old boy could muster up, "This is my Oma. She was so very special, and you have to know that she loved and cared for all of us." What a final tribute to a life well-lived, a life defined by her daily love and care for others. With no words left to speak, I thought to myself as we walked away from the grave site, *we will miss you, but those marks you left on our souls will never be erased. Goodbye, my faithful companion.*

A Brief Reflection

Erik Erikson, renowned for his theories on the stages of psycho-social development, believed that the last phases of a "good life" are completed with a deep, well-defined sense of integrity. For Erikson, integrity implied the acceptance of a life well-lived. So fitting for Jeanette. She lived and served humbly, purposefully, and always with great care and compassion. One of the questions I struggled periodically with was that of healing. I wanted her to be healed, I wanted God to heal her, and I wanted her to want that too, but she didn't. She believed, saw, and experienced the power of healing throughout her lifetime, yet that wasn't ever a request she brought before the Lord. One time, while sitting in service, the pastor made an altar call for those who were sick in body to come forward that we might pray for their healing. I believed in that moment that God could heal her; I really sensed that she was to go forward to be healed. So I asked her if she wanted to go to the altar. Her reply both shocked me and (maybe, not initially) humored me. She said, "Why would I go? I don't need to be prayed for. If you want to be prayed for, you go!"

Maybe she couldn't see the necessity because of her confused state of mind, or maybe she saw with greater clarity than I could. She was satisfied that the Lord had and was continuing to accomplish His work in her life as planned. No mistakes. No miscalculations. There was no despair, hopelessness, loss of purpose, or loss of any other virtues[52] she had acquired over the course of her lifetime. The issue of life and death were both resolved in her Hope of a continued future in Christ. Jeanette had lived a good life surrounded by people she loved and who loved her back. She accomplished more in her life, surely, than she could have conceived as a young girl growing up poor in Chattanooga, Tennessee. She had *become*. According to

---

52 Erikson assumes that a crisis occurs at each stage of development. Successful completion of each stage results generally in a healthy personality and the acquisition of basic virtues. Basic virtues are strengths which the ego can use to resolve subsequent crises. He envisioned these eight stages in contrast to their competitors. They are: (1) Trust vs Mistrust (ages, infancy); (2) Autonomy vs Shame (early childhood); (3) Initiative vs Guilt (Play age, 3-5); (4) Industry vs Inferiority (School age, 5 – 12); (5) Ego Identity vs Role Confusion (Adolescence, 12-18) (6) Intimacy vs Isolation (Young adult); (7) Generativity vs Stagnation (Adulthood, 40-65 plus); (8) Ego Integrity vs Despair (Maturity, 65-on). Saul McLeod, "Erik Erikson," Simply Psychology, 2008, accessed Dec. 2015, http://www.simplypsychology.org/Erik-Erikson.html.

Erikson's evaluation, she successfully completed her final stage here on earth, resulting in her acquisition of Ego Integrity with wisdom as the chief virtue acquired. The Word of God says it like this: "Well done, my good and faithful servant."

Chapter 10

The God Who Sees Me: A Visitation

"For still the vision awaits its appointed time;
it hastens to the end – it will not lie.
If it seems slow, wait for it;
it will surely come;
it will not delay."
—Habakkuk 2:3 (ESV)

Probably the most significant and deeply lasting event that occurred in this whole process came after the end, after the funeral, after we left her buried in a grave, after everyone left, and after we returned to a home emptied of my beloved wife. It is in this final chapter that I share with you that very personal and life-changing event which took place the day after Jeanette's graveside service. Naturally, some will be skeptical. I only ask you take the time, as I have for the last year and a half, to measure this account in terms of who our loving Lord is and what the Word of God says about this and other interventions of the Holy Spirit. By

233

now you are probably asking yourself, *what is all this about? Why all the delay?* The simple answer is fear. I recognize that by sharing this event I risk my present and future reputation; yet, this occurrence was more real to me than any other spiritual event I've been privileged to experience. Call it what you may: a vision, special revelation, or simply a personal visit of the Holy Spirit. I call it *El-Roi*. For, like Hagar, God allowed me to see Him seeing me.

In Genesis chapter sixteen, Sarai, desperate for a child, requests her husband take a young servant girl named Hagar as a wife so they can have a child. When Hagar conceived, the relationship between the two women became greatly distressed. Sarai, full of contempt, wanted her gone and "dealt harshly with her." As a result, Hagar fled from her, running into the desert. The scene seems almost desperate as Hagar lays down, defeated and exhausted, next to a spring of water, most likely crying out for some kind of intervention. In response to her cry, a most amazing thing occurred. The God of this great world not only heard her cries, but looked on her anguish and saw her. I'm not sure what it is about grief that leaves us running for the desert to hide, all the while wanting nothing more than some kind of divine intervention: to be seen, to be acknowledged and to be validated by our Heavenly Father. Hagar was gifted with such an *El-Roi. The God Who Sees* made a point to let her see Him seeing her. And, that is what *The God Who Sees* did for me.

I have had only one other supernatural intervention through a vision. I was 11 years old and going through a very difficult time with my family. My mother suffered very serious emotional and mental struggles. She was severely depressed and often threatened suicide in order to get the attention she needed from a troubled relationship with my dad. One night I could endure it no longer. If she wasn't going to do it, then I would! Afflicted by her disease, I left my farm house in the middle of the night to make good on her threats of death. I headed for our cattle pond. Even in the darkness of night, the pond was bright red, the color of the earth from which it was dug. Peaceful. Untouched by the tumultuous times which surrounded it. That night, I was determined that this man-made pond, purposed to be a resting place for our cattle who sought refuge from the scorching summer heat, would be my last resting place. My peace. My refuge from the scorching heat of a pain-filled life. A perfect—even ironic— end to a most imperfect existence. *Certainly,* I thought, *this will end my pain.*

I was a boy with a heavy load of troubles. As I walked across our small forty-acre farm, my attention was drawn to a large slate rock which sat in the middle of our main pasture. I had seen the rock many times, but on that moonlit night, it was as if I was viewing the rock for the first time. The moon beams shone brightly on its slate, giving it a magical appearance as air particles glistened and danced lightly all around the rock, thus creating for this country boy a spectacular, mystical sight. I was instinctively drawn to the rock, when suddenly a voice spoke within me—a voice I remember to this day. *Kneel and pray.* I obeyed. Immediately I saw fast-moving scenes. They weren't

> *El-Roi, The God Who Sees, made a point to let her see Him seeing her. And, that is what The God Who Sees did for me.*

externally visible; it was as if they were memories being replayed in my mind, but they were not my memories. They were images implanted on my mind's heart. It was as if the Lord said, "Take a look at what I have planned for you, and DO NOT miss it!"

Through the Holy Spirit's intervening vision, I saw myself in numerous scenes. In one, I was dressed up in nice pants and a coat (a desire of a poor, farm boy's heart; in fact, my siblings and I would often watch passenger trains fly by on the tracks beside our home, observing those of wealth in the dinner car and unrealistically fantasizing that someday we could be so fortunate). In another, I saw myself speaking to groups of soldiers, just like I did years later when I was serving as a military chaplain. The Spirit then took me to another scene: a party with lots of food in an environment of joy and friendship—a scene so contrary to the life of poverty and invisibility which I had experienced. Maybe that is the greater significance of God's intervention that night. It happened to me—an insignificant and forgotten child of 16 kids in a large, blended family during the bleakest, most hopeless time in American history, *The Great Depression*. What possible significance could *that kid* have in God's greater plan for His Kingdom?

There was one last detail that never left that eleven-year-old boy. It was the image of a beautiful lady whom I now know to be Jeanette. Years later, when I first met Jeanette as a high school student, my mind went back to that slate rock scene. I told my friend after first meeting her, "That is the person I will marry someday." He laughed and teasingly replied, "Are you kidding me? There is no way she would ever have you!" I knew better...I "saw" better. And a year later, I married the girl of my vision.

Whatever happened to me in the summer of 1941 left such a deep impression that when I left that slate rock I was determined to find a way to be that person and to experience the great plans the Lord had waiting me. Throughout my life, I would revisit that vision as a point of reference during times of trials and sorrows. In so doing, the Lord would remind me of those promises which even to this day I treasure.

That event with the Lord and the one I will now share will never be doubted in my heart. Yet I write it cautiously and purposefully, so that those who read the vision may run with vision (Habakkuk 2:2). For though we may, at times, wait for the Lord's Word to find us, see us, and reveal itself, I know and bear witness that it will surely come and not delay. This vision is a reminder—a promise — that the Eternal Lord cares personally for each of us, for you and for me. He cared when I was a distraught child at the young age of 11; He cares for this husband, father, and grandfather trying to find meaning after the loss of a long-term life and ministry companion, and He cares for you no matter how great your struggle might be. Now, share with me in this final visitation which moves us from our present journey to *beyond...* .

The Vision Awaits its Appointed Time

I spent so much of my life caring for her that leaving her in that casket, alone, seemed a betrayal of my heart. My need to protect her and keep her safely with me overwhelmed me. I was helpless as my world seemed to be without form and void. A great darkness hung over the face of the deepest parts of me. No order existed in my heart or mind as I made my way, with the kids beside me, back to our home in Georgia. The drive home seemed to last forever. I thought the weighted-ness of our collective grief would suffocate me before we could return home. I just wanted to be out of the confinements of that car and the heavy presence therein. I wanted to be home, in our home. Away from the right things to say and the parade of misshapen smiles and hugs. I felt like a robot, mechanical and functional, but absent of self, as if my spirit had somehow disconnected from my body. That evening my family tried to comfort me, but I was beyond the reaches of their comfort and care. Peace was so far from my heart; I was travailing.

I went to bed early but was unable to sleep. That next morning I was a complete wreck. It was as if everything within me had been emptied. I was all dried up, unable to even cry out to the Lord for help. How He could even help me at this point was beyond my understanding. She was gone and all was hopelessly lost. Jonne finally said to me, "Dad, you must go to bed and get some rest. You look terrible." So I excused myself and headed for the room where Jeanette had died a few days earlier. I just wanted to lay on her bed and be near her in some way. Without thinking, as if compelled, I found myself reaching over and touching her spot—maybe out of a need to confirm that she was really gone; maybe to keep me connected to a reality that was still too surreal to own; or, maybe out of a need to just connect with her in any way possible, even if it wasn't sensible. As I lay there, a wave of reality settled in my heart and a breaking occurred. I began to sob openly and uncontrollably. I cried out to my Lord in desperation for Him to step into my experience and make me well. Hearing my cries, Jonne twice came to my bedroom door to see if I was okay. I wasn't okay; okay was so far from where I was. I was sinking into a dark abyss and crying out for the Lord to somehow deliver me. Yet, needing to give her some kind of response, I offered her up a "thanks for caring" and sent her away. Hesitantly and obediently, she left me to wrestle with my anguish and grief.

I was overtly desperate. I pleaded with the Lord to come to me. I needed relief, death, or just a simple sign. I even pleaded with him to send me a sign of His nearness. *Just move the curtains; let me know you are here. Anything! I need you so badly, Lord.* Then something happened. The curtains moved! I was stunned, momentarily, until our faithful dog Skipper came out from behind them. Dismayed, I thought, *Oh God! Is this all I will get?* I was so desperate. I began to cry even louder, "Oh, God! I do no ask you to bring Jeanette back. That would be contrary to your Word. Yet, I plead with you. Give me some assurance that she made it safely into your divine presence."

Like a parent anxiously waiting by the phone for their child to assure them he or she had safely arrived at a distant destination, I waited inconsolably for a "call" that could not possibly come. Getting nowhere in this epic battle of my soul, I broke. Fully submitted to the truth before me, I conceded. *I'm just going to give it all to you, Lord. I surrender. Whatever you want, I am ready to receive.* Within seconds I felt the room lighten up a little. I looked at the drapes to see if it was the sun shining through them. I checked the clock; it was 1:30 p.m. What happened next forever changed me. I heard a voice softly say, "I am here. What do you want?" I thought to myself, *this cannot be. Is this really her?* Naturally, my clinical training and experiences have made me somewhat suspicious of these kinds of supernatural experiences. I looked around the room at the different pictures and the clock on the wall to assure myself that I was awake and not in some dream-like state. Not convinced, I pinched my arm. *I must be asleep.* Again, I heard the voice speak, this time sternly, impatiently, "I am here. What do you want?" *Okay,* I thought, *Lord this has got to be something very special from you. I know I am saved. I am not subject to irrational behavior like hearing voices; I will just go ahead and assume this is Jeanette and accept it in faith.*

> *"This is not about me. This is about your relationship with our Father who felt your pain and heard your plea."*

The voice sounded like "Old Jeanette," my healthy earthly companion for so many years, not "Sick Jeanette," who had just passed away. Still cautious, I asked, "Jeanette, is that you?"

She replied, "Yes, the Father sent me. What do you want?" Before I could respond, she cautioned, "This is not about me. This is about your relationship with our Father who felt your pain and heard your plea."

As I remember, I said, "I understand, but can I ask you something?"

She said, "Of course, that is why the Father sent me."

Compelled by a lifetime of being her spiritual covering, I asked the question most pressing on my heart, "Did you make it home okay?"

"I did."

Immediately, I felt a great release from the heaviness that had weighed on me since the funeral. I broke into uncontrollable crying again. Relieved of my burden, I could finally lift up my heart to the Lord: *Oh, Lord, my precious one is okay. She is safe at home with you, our Lord!* After a few minutes, I collected myself and asked her a second question, "How did it happen? How did you get there from here?"

Her response felt like every other conversation we had ever had, so natural and unforced, "Well, it is like waking from surgery. You are awakened and hear voices. One said, 'Welcome to Paradise.'"

This beautiful, extra-worldly experience was too great to be fully realized in the moment. At times I was certain I was experiencing some kind of mental break, a delusional moment; so I evaluated myself by periodically checking the clock. Finally, I convinced myself that, yes, this was really happening. Humbly, I said in my heart, *I will not doubt you again, Lord.*

As our conversation continued, Jeanette occasionally reminded me that this was not about her, but about my relationship with the Heavenly Father. With that settled, I continued to ask other questions. Every time my question reached farther than the parameters given for our conversation, she would check me with the same phrases: "This is about your relationship with the Father," "You know better than to ask me that," or "Let's not go there."

I knew this to be the Jeanette I had known all those years; she always kept our conversations within the boundaries of reasonableness, even as we talked out the most important and pressing issues in our lives. She seldom discussed matters just to appease her curiosity.

Having a growing sense of certainty about this encounter, I knew it must be ordered by my Heavenly Father. It is His very nature to personally care for one of His lost sheep afflicted by a broken heart. I was so humbled that He would allow Jeanette to visit with me and grateful that this special encounter did not come by way of a newly revised Jeanette; rather, she came to me as her truest self with all of her unique personality traits, nuances, and personal history. Knowing I had limited access to her newfound knowledge, I enquired, "Can I ask you another question?"

"Go ahead."

"What is paradise like?"

"Oh, it is wonderful! You would not want to miss coming here. Our human minds could not describe with words what God has waiting for us here. Everyone is so beautiful, loving each other, praising our Lord. I am so happy."

Confounded by the knowledge that she was already in paradise, I asked, "Why are you there?" Her answer shocked me since I would often comfort grieving families explaining that their loved one left this world and woke up in the arms of Jesus.

"I am here being prepared to be the Bride of Christ."

Captivated, I responded, "Jeanette, that is something. I have always understood the story of the *Ten Virgins* in terms of the Second Coming. But it makes sense. We all must be prepared for that grand wedding feast with our Lord and Savior."

"Of course."

Eventually, I asked the most obvious question, "How are we being allowed this conversation, if you are in Paradise and I am still stuck on earth?"

Her response made perfect, eternal sense. "Our Lord is master of the One Kingdom; Earth and Heaven are part of that One Kingdom. We are separated only in terms of His mission. We are both still in His One Kingdom."

I quickly responded, "But this earth is so troubled. There is so much evil."

"Remember, it is His One Kingdom. While there may be evil, it is still His good earth."

Stunned and intrigued, her answered stirred up more questions than answers within me. "Why would you say that?"

She spoke so honestly and rationally. Her answers included facts of time and places on earth. "It is God's good earth. Had I not been there (earth), I could not be here (Paradise). You remember, I was saved and filled with the Holy Spirit at the Alton Park Church of God in 1946 (two years before we were married). Had I not had that earthly experience, I would never have the joy of being here."

I thought to myself, *this is real. I would have never thought of that illustration on my own.* The Father was not only comforting me with spiritual presence, but with the factual assurances of events that brought fact and faith into total unity. Beyond theological questions, I ventured into more personal questions and confessions despite her reminders that the visit was not about her. I knew this would be my last chance to confess some things that I had carried with me for years. "Jeanette, I have always felt guilty about going into the military and taking you from your home in Chattanooga, especially from your mom and dad whom you loved so dearly. We moved so many times. I have felt guilty not giving you the stability you deserved."

Her response was so typical of my Jeanette. She said, "Don't be silly. Do you remember when you met me in Bremerhaven, Germany?" (In 1953, as a low-ranked airman in the Air Force, I brought Jeanette over on a tourist visa for six months.)

"Yes."

"When I got off the ship and we got on the train for Landsberg, I remember looking around at all those different people with their different clothing styles. Looking out the window of the train and seeing all those new sights, I thought to myself, *I have married a man that will show me God's whole earth.*"

In that sacred moment, I realized that her words released me from all that guilt I had carried so unnecessarily for years. We had together experienced the vastness of this good earth. We have seen and experienced some of the most beautiful aspects this world has to offer and have seen the most depraved and sorrowful places that exist. Our journey took us around the world. How could we have foreseen such a magnificent journey in our runaway marriage?

Wanting our time together to last, I asked more questions, "What do you hold most precious of your years on earth?"

"Of course, being a mother."

"Why?"

"I was given the joy of raising our kids."

"Could you tell me how you felt about our kids, David, Jonne, and Dale?"

She replied matter-of-factly, "David was my little man. I loved watching him walk, play little games, and share the many stories of his activities. Jonne was so pretty. I loved making her clothes and watching her walk around the room admiring herself. And, Dale, the little stinker, always looked for trouble. He was so small, but so sweet."

I was amazed to discover that the Lord's intervention is both of faith and fact. This revelation showed me, and hopefully others, that those important life events such as salvation, baptism in the Holy Spirit, marriage, children, etc. will forever be incorporated into our heavenly body and state. I will leave it up to the Lord to explain to us how we can be new creatures while fully ourselves—memories and personal history intact.

Curiosity fully heightened, I pushed into areas, apparently from her responses, that were not at all relevant to the purpose of her visit. I told her a little about the funeral and the graveside service. Then I asked her, "Do you remember anything about your funeral? Lots of people came to honor you."

She stated in typical Jeanette fashion, "You know better than to worry about that. The funeral was about us, not you and the Father. Don't ask those questions. I came straight here to be in this

245

wonderful place, Paradise." Appropriately rebuked and humored, I thought, *typical Jeanette*.

Jeanette always told me not to worry about her burial. She wasn't planning on being in that grave. She had a greater vision than mere death; she planned to live eternally. As the conversation began to weaken, she reminded me a final time, "This is not about me. I am okay in this wonderful place awaiting to be the Bride of Christ. This is about you and your relationship with the Father. He heard your cry, He feels your pain, and He sent me only as His messenger to bring comfort to your heart."

While I cannot recall every detail of our visit, in my heart I do remember how steeped in scripture many of her answers were. She referenced passages such as 1 Corinthians 2:9: "Eye has not seen, nor ear heard…the things which God has prepared for those who love Him." I cannot say with certainty that she quoted the entire passage, but she definitely quoted portions of it. Several times various passages from the Psalms would be integrated into her responses: "Blessed is he, whose help is the God of Jacob…the Maker of heaven and earth, the sea, and everything in them" (Ps. 146), and "God is my refuge, my portion, in the land of the living" (Ps. 142). Even the scriptures referenced in her conversation seemed to fit with her constant refrain: "This is not about me; it's about you and your relationship with the Lord."

Near the close, she exhorted me to "live again and love again." With that and the joy I felt at that moment, I knew the reason for this experience was to bring a measure of closure. I genuinely thanked her for those many years with me and the kids. I thanked her for all the things she had done for us and so many others. She simply responded, "I am okay; I am home. This is not about me; it is about the Father's love for you, His child."

I felt her fading from me. My tears flowed freely, openly and full of thanksgiving like a child whose parent had just fulfilled the passions of their hearts. In that moment, I found the strength to offer up thoughts of joy and celebration at the news: *Jeanette is home; she has now journeyed into this other part of God's Kingdom with the redeemed.* I felt fully grateful having her as my lifelong companion, the driving force of my journey, through years of family, life, and ministry. Though grieved, I was wholly satisfied by this last encounter with her, which I will carry me until that time I join her for all eternity in God's One Kingdom. As she faded, all I could say was, "Goodbye Jeanette," and "Thank you, Lord, for you are, indeed, wonderful."

I looked at the clock, again. I had been in this spiritual dimension for about 40 minutes. I was so amazed at God's response to my deep loss and grief. I lay there, thinking, *What a Savior! What a Loving Father! What a Comforting Holy Spirit!* I knew what had happened to me was so contrary to the way I generally lived. We were rational and academic, not given to such extraordinary experiences. Yes, we are Pentecostal and recognize the sovereign power of this Almighty God to do above and beyond what we are able to humanly conceive. Yet knowing that our God is always present and always hears our cries for help, we seldom *expect* Him to personally intervene with such a powerful and loving response. He never fails to see us. He never fails to come to our aid. He is ever present, willing, able, and always on our side. He comforts us in the most unique and gentle ways: "This is not about me; I have arrived safely." And He pursues us beyond the borders and limitation of our human rationale: "This is about *your relationship* with our Loving Father."

After a few moments of collecting myself, I finally left my bedroom. Jonne and Dale were sitting in the living room. They knew something special had happened; it showed in my countenance. For, just as His assurances lifted and changed the countenance of Hannah in First Samuel, so He lifted and changed mine. The psalmist named Him *Rumn Rosh*, "the lifter of my head" (Ps. 3). In my heart and like so many other biblical characters who had a life-changing encounter with God, I named Him, too. I named him *El Roi*, the God who sees me, and *Rumn Rosh*, the lifter of my head (Ps. 3:3). For my Abba Father heard my cry and attuned himself to my need. Then He looked on me and lifted my hanging head.

As I recounted the details of *my* encounter to the kids, they were amazed at the great works of the Lord. They understood that this visitation wasn't about morbid curiosity with the afterlife or even my inability to let go of Jeanette. The significance of my encounter was about a Heavenly Father who greatly loves his children…who greatly loves me. This is the Abba Father who came to me when I was in such a desperate state of need. He saw me and heard me; He came near to me. And He alone satisfied my dry and empty soul!

Not needing any confirmations, the Lord graciously gave them to me anyway. They didn't come from prominent men or any of the other expected places. Rather, God chose an unusual voice, yet wholly trustworthy: my granddaughter. My granddaughter, Rachel, had what she calls a vision at only three years old, following the funeral of her Aunt Virginia. Now nine years old, she responded to my encounter with all the spiritual maturity of a seasoned theologian and yet the innocence of an insightful child. She said with certainty and conviction, "Opa, you know that once you have a vision, it can never go away from your mind. The Lord won't let it leave!" She continued, "As you think about your vision, you will see even more things (I imagine she meant details) that you may have missed or forgotten." Whether this budding theologian was right or not about visions, I believed her. God has a way of speaking to us in the most unexpected places. I'm learning how to listen for Him in those places, to embrace ideas and knowledge outside my previously gained understanding of God's One Kingdom, and to more and more see this earth, wrought with sinful persons and deeds, as still God's good earth. The good news is that none of us would ever be given the joy of receiving him into our hearts were it not, as Jeanette stated, "For our good earth experience." That is my resolve, to have a good earth experience even in a war-torn world. For God is an ever present help, always pursuing and intervening on our behalf.

Jeanette's journey through the land and language of Alzheimer's was transformational for all those who, to the best of their ability, remained in the journey. For they too were called to discard all their baggage in order to journey well. Through this cleansing, our Lord assisted us in returning to the most sacred aspect of our life: our relationship with him and with each other. While our journey toward death was often confusing and painful, it was also cleansing. And in this holy, cleansing process, that which was sacred, those deeds written into the "Book of Life" were retained and will be incorporated in us as we become the redeemed, glorified children of God, who are being prepared *in paradise* to become, like all the redeemed, the Bride of Christ! That is why I could lay down my baggage and can now call forth others to lay theirs down with me. For as the prophet Habakkuk recorded, the recipient of the vision must run with it. That is my new journey: to finish the final leg of my journey revealing the personal, intimate love of God and calling others to share in the *Sacramental Cleansing* which releases us to experience the vastness of God's love. Having likewise received the vision, you must also run with it in whatever way the Lord reveals it to you— whether expanding your "inclusive" church ministries to encompass homebound individuals and families or simply your personal care of the sick (physically, intellectually, or mentally), the naked, the imprisoned, the poor, and the homeless. Wherever it takes you, I assure you, it is a worthwhile journey. Yet let me caution you. The message of the vision isn't a leisurely journey. It is wrought with great pain and sacrifice, yet its cost is outweighed by the bountiful blessings gleaned along the way. For those of you willing to persevere and remain on the journey (run with the vision), God's promise is for you to be cleansed by your sacrament of care for those who need your presence through whatever lands God call them and you to. But you must travel light, casting all your cares and baggage (ministry, relationships, successes and losses, titles and labels, inflated egos and self-hatred) on Him, for *El-Roi* "cares about you [with deepest affection, and watches over you very carefully]" (1 Pt. 5:7b AMP).

May you journey well... .

Bibliography

Barth, Karl. The Humanity of God: Essay Three, trans. Thomas Wieser. Louisville: Richmond, VA: Westminster John Knox Press, 1960. https://archive.org/details/TheHumanityOf-God-KarlBarth

Bonhoeffer, Deitrich. "Who Am I?" International Bonhoeffer Society English Language Section, 1945. Accessed 11 November 2015, www.dbonhoeffer.org/who-was-db2.htm

Chapman, Gary. "Marriage: Covenant or Contract?" Lifeway. HomeLife, 3 January 2014. Accessed 8 August 2015. www.lifeway.com/Article/HomeLife-Marriage-Covenant-or-Contract.

Foster, David K. "Covenant: The Heart of the Marriage Mystery." Focus on the Family. n.d. Accessed 15 August 2015. www.focusonthefamily.com

Gopnik, Alison. "Is our Identity in Intellect, Memory or Moral Character?" The Wall Street Journal. September 9, 2015. Accessed November 21, 2015. www.wsj.com/articles/is-our-identity-in-intellect-memory-or-moral-character-1441812784

Hahn, Scott. "Contract versus Covenant." Outlook. Worldview Publications, February 2002. Accessed 15 August 2015. www.worldviewpublications.org/outlook/archive/main.php?EDITION=043

McLeod, Saul. "Erik Erikson." Simply Psychology. 2008. Accessed December 2015, www.simiplypsychology.org/Erik-Erikson.html,

Nouwen, Henri. The Wounded Healer: Ministry in Contemporary Society. New York: Doubleday Dell Publishing Group, Inc, 1972.

O'Brien, Greg. On Pluto: Inside the Mind of Alzheimer's. Brewster, MA: Codfish Press, 2014.

Ridderbos, Herman. "The Epistle of Paul to the Churches of Galatia." Grand Rapids: Eerdmans, 1953. Bible Research. Accessed 8 August 2015. www.bible-researcher.com/covenant.html

Shenk, David. "What is Alzheimer's?" A Quick Look at Alzheimer's. Accessed November 2015. www.aboutalz.org

Singer, Megan. "2013 State of the Climate: Record-breaking Super Typhoon Haiyan." Climate.gov. July 13, 2014. Accessed 22 January 2016. www.climate.gov

Strohminger, Nina and Shaun Nichols, "The Essential Moral Self. Psychological Science," Cognition, 131 (2014): 159-171. Accessed November 21, 2015. www.elsevier.com/locate/COGNIT

Wynkoop, Mildred Bangs. A Theology of Love: The Dynamic of Wesleyanism. Kansas City, Missouri: Beacon Hill Press of Kansas City, 1972.

Recommended Resources

Books/articles

Callone, et.al. A Caregiver's Guide to Alzheimer's Disease: 300 Tips for Making Life Easier. New York: Demos Medical Publications, 2006.

Coste, Joanne Koenig. Learning to Speak Alzheimer's: A Groundbreaking Approach for Everyone Dealing with the Disease. New York: Houghton Mifflin Company, 2003.

Gopnik, Alison. "Is our Identity in Intellect, Memory or Moral Character?" The Wall Street Journal. September 9, 2015. Accessed November 21, 2015. www.wsj.com/articles/is-our-identity-in-intellect-memory-or-moral-character-1441812784

Kessler, Lauren. Finding Life in the Land of Alzheimer's: One Daughter's Hopeful Story. New York: Penguin Books, 2007.

"Understanding Alzheimer's Disease: What you need to know." National Institute on Aging. NIH Publication No. 11-5441, June 2011.

Nouwen, Henri J.M. A Spirituality of Caregiving, ed, John S. Mogabgab . Nashville: Upper Room Books, 2011.

O'Brien, Greg. On Pluto: Inside the Mind of Alzheimer's. Brewster, MA: Codfish Press, 2014.

Phelps, Rick & Gary Joseph LeBlanc. While I Still Can...One Man's Journey through Early Onset Alzheimer's Disease.

s.n., 2012.

Strohminger, Nina and Shaun Nichols, "The Essential Moral Self. Psychological Science," Cognition, 131 (2014): 159-171. Accessed November 21, 2015. www.elsevier.com/locate/COGNIT

Wynkoop, Mildred Bangs. A Theology of Love: The Dynamic of Wesleyanism. Kansas City, Missouri: Beacon Hill Press of Kansas City, 1972.

Websites

Alzheimer's Association, www.alz.org/facts/

Alzheimer's Disease Education and Referral Center (ADEAR), www.nia.hih.gov/Alzheimers

Alzheimer's Foundation of America, www.alzfdn.org

Alzheimer's Reading Room (A site providing updated information and support for individuals and families experiencing Alzheimer's), www.alzheimersreadingroom.com

A Quick Look at Alzheimer's (video series on Alzheimer's disease), www.aboutalz.org

Eldercare Locator, www.eldercare.gov

IF YOU'RE A FAN OF THIS BOOK, PLEASE TELL OTHERS

■ Write about it on your blog and on Twitter and on your Facebook and LinkedIn pages.

■ Suggest it to friends.

■ When you're in a bookstore, ask them if they carry the book. The book is available through all major distributors, so any bookstore that does not have it can easily order it.

■ Write a positive review on www.amazon.com.

■ Send my publisher, HigherLife Publishing (media@ahigherlife.com), suggestions about websites, conferences, and events you know of where this book could be offered.

■ Purchase additional copies to give away as gifts.

ALSO BY ROBERT CRICK

Outside the Gates: The Need for Theology, History, and Practice of Chaplaincy Ministries

The great task before Christian workers, chaplains in particular, is to find a way to work within the systems of this world in order to redeem and sanctify those systems in the authority of our Lord, Jesus Christ, who sends them. Chaplains are present in some of the darkest, most impoverished, oppressed, and immoral places on this earth. Their mission is very clear: to be present with the brokenhearted and needy, while working with and within the systems that affect the lives of those they seek to help.

Outside the Gates is available at **outsidethegates.org**.